PERILOUS PILLS

PROTECTING YOURSELF
FROM FLUOROQUINOLONE INJURY

MARILYN BEARDSLEY HEISE

PERILOUS PILLS

Published by
BIRDSEED, LLC

ISBN 978-1-7333905-0-7

The purpose of this book is informational and educational
and any advice therein is not to be considered medical
advice or treatment and is not intended to replace the
professional services of a physician. The author does not
endorse linked websites or resources as they are provided
merely as a service to readers.

*To do no harm going forward, we
must be able to learn from the
harm we have already done.*

DR. MARTY MAKARY
SURGEON, JOHNS HOPKINS HOSPITAL

*There is no more powerful force
than an informed consumer.*

ALEX M. AZAR II
U.S. SECRETARY OF HEALTH AND HUMAN SERVICES

CONTENTS

PROLOGUE

IT ALL STARTED for me with a minor sinus infection and taking a prescription called Levaquin, a fluoroquinolone antibiotic. Severe stiffness and pain came on suddenly in legs, ankles, hips, arms, wrists and shoulders as I awoke one morning and was so disabling, I was barely able to roll out of bed. I discovered later that I had also suffered a tear in a shoulder's rotator cuff. It turned out that I was suffering from an all-body tendon inflammation called tendonitis. That happened several days after I had taken the medicine prescribed by my doctor. I was convinced that this sudden painful and disabling condition had to be the result of taking that drug.

As I spoke with friends about my experience, I began to hear other stories of bodily harm, sometimes permanent, from taking this particular drug. The internet revealed hundreds of tales of healthy, active people who had had debilitating experiences after taking these medications. Organizations and help groups were active and thriving. The manufacturer of Levaquin was facing thousands of lawsuits brought by injured patients. The government's Food and Drug Administration had slapped a black box warning on Levaquin cautioning about a multitude of possible dangers.

When I went back to read the information flier given by the pharmacy with my prescription, I saw in bold letters that taking Levaquin could quite possibly cause rupture of the Achilles tendon. Public Citizen's Health Research Group, publisher of *Worst Pills, Best Pills*, had deemed Levaquin a Limited Use Drug.

What was going on here?

Why were there so many people being hurt and disabled by these prescription medications? How do these damaging drugs get on the market? Are prescriptions from your doctor safe to take? Are these drugs given to patients in hospitals and other institutions? Why are doctors prescribing pills that can cause such harm? Is anyone doing anything about this?

I became alarmed and as a journalist, I thought I should investigate further.

This journey researching fluoroquinolones has taken more than six years. It has yielded hundreds of sources of information. It has revealed a robust internet that teems with stories told by victims about their heartbreaking experiences after they took these particular pills. With most doctors denying that their patients had been injured and scoffing at the suggestion, it appeared that the internet had become a last resort for victims crying out for help.

I discovered that the U.S.'s regulatory agency is remarkably unreliable, biased and slow to respond to reports of drug injury. Research exposed a pharmaceutical industry that was making billions of dollars from sales of fluoroquinolones as they became among one of the most prescribed meds in the world. It was disturbing to see that sales continued even as injuries and life-long disabilities had been reported for nearly 40 years since they had been introduced to the marketplace. Drug companies, it appeared, are driven by huge profits, leading them to undertake questionable, even dangerous, promotion and sales practices. Hospitals were freely giving these antibiotics as a preventative rather than a cure.

And yes, the doctor's office had been invaded, too. The influence of pharmaceutical companies, regulations, restrictions, and burnout have taken a toll on physicians and the patients in their care.

I have been appalled, astounded and angered by what I have learned. I hope the reader will experience similar reactions upon reading this book and will advocate rigorously for change and awareness. This volume is filled with revelations about the manufacture, regulation and practice of prescribing a class of antibiotics that has injured hundreds of thousands of individuals who trusted their doctors and the medical system to heal and not harm them.

It has become my mission, my passion, to create awareness and warn patients and their loved ones of the risks associated with taking fluoroquinolones as well as to reveal the larger story behind them.

HARMS AND HURTS

*If this toxicity can happen to a
young and healthy person like
me, it can happen to anyone.*

JOHN FRATTI

AS I WAS going through the lengthy quest of being referred from doctor to doctor to determine why I had
that disabling stiffness and muscular pain after taking
Levaquin, I began sharing my story with friends. With
profound amazement, I quickly discovered that there
were at least ten others who had also experienced an
adverse reaction to Levaquin or a medication in this
same class of antibiotics. Others said someone they
knew had had a similar experience resulting from taking
these drugs. Here are just a few of their painful stories:

Joanie had been prescribed Levaquin that resulted
in severe "plantar fasciitis," a very painful heel and
bottom of the foot injury. She was unable to walk for
weeks, wear shoes for months, and only fully recovered two years later. (Plantar fascia is the flat ligament
band that connects your heel bone to your toes and
supports the arch of your foot. Fasciitis occurs when

there are micro tears in the ligament, one of the possible side effects of fluoroquinolone use, I was soon to find out.)

Marybeth, an active 69-year-old, walked three miles daily and exercised at a Curves facility in spite of being a controlled Type 1 diabetic and taking medication for high blood pressure and thyroid disease. She had two rounds of the antibiotic Azithromycin for an upper respiratory infection, but severe and recurring sore throats two months later sent her back to her internist. He wrote a prescription for Levaquin, noting that "this is the gold standard, a last-ditch effort." He said he was taking it himself to alleviate a cough acquired on a recent trip to China. It sounded like it should be safe.

Nevertheless, after taking two pills, she began having severe pain in both legs and had difficulty walking. She took another pill prior to phoning the doctor, who said to stop taking it immediately. He prescribed ice packs and Aleve. With severe pain continuing and both legs swollen and bruised, Marybeth went back to her physician, who referred her to an orthopedic surgeon. He confirmed a diagnosis of ruptured Achilles tendons in both ankles. Surgery was the usual treatment, she was told, but that "complete healing would be difficult."

Marybeth declined surgery because of her diabetic dependence and the risk seemed to outweigh the benefit. She was fitted with knee-high orthopedic boots and wore them for two months, then transitioned to regular shoes with lifts and use of a cane. She also acquired plantar fasciitis, which continued for many months.

During a follow up interview years after her incident, she reported continued weakness in both legs, said she didn't walk properly, had difficulty climbing stairs, and wore special shoes. Since our first interview, she has had knee surgery to repair two rips in the meniscus, a possible result of the Achilles tendon ruptures years before, she was told. (The meniscus is a rubbery C-shaped disc that cushions your knee and helps keep the joint steady. When torn, the knee becomes wobbly and prevents the joint from working properly.)

Betsy felt sick and went to the emergency room at a local hospital on Christmas Day, where she was diagnosed with pneumonia. She was given Levaquin, sent home, and developed a raging case of hives. The doctor thought she was having "an allergic reaction to the medicine" and asked her to return to the hospital. The hives calmed down but left large patches of red skin. While at the hospital, however, Betsy's nurse related an identical story of what had happened to one of her co-workers who had taken Levaquin!

It was not only friends who seemed to have encountered these Levaquin adverse events. While I was telling a podiatrist about my experience, he said, "Oh, yes. I had one of those, too." He offered to tell me his story, then had second thoughts and declined.

A friend referred me to a dentist who used to be an avid tennis player, but after taking both Levaquin and Cipro, he suffered bilateral tendon ruptures in both knees requiring surgery. "I can no longer move fast enough to compete in tennis" he told me. "My tennis days are over, now I'm just happy I can walk."

I called Mike, referred by a friend, who was prescribed Levaquin by his physician when he was ill and pneumonia was suspected. His doctor called a prescription for Levaquin "the silver bullet." After a week to ten days, Mike developed a painful meniscus tear in his knee (he had had one years before) for no apparent reason. Although Mike said he can't prove it came from Levaquin, he sees no other answer.

One of the most severe and frightening encounters with this drug, told to me by a retired physician, was about his practice partner's son. The son, normal in every way including psychologically, was a practicing doctor of medicine in Mexico. He took Levaquin for an ailment, suffered hallucinations, and two days later jumped from a bridge, killing himself.

After hearing these worrisome stories just from casually talking to friends and friends of friends, I became alarmed and began exploring further. Newspapers, magazines, books, the internet…all were chock full of similar medical stories. It was hard to believe. How could a widely used drug be doing all this harm without restraints and apparently being prescribed under approval from a government agency that was to protect the public?

AS I BEGAN researching, I discovered that Levaquin was manufactured by Johnson & Johnson (J&J). It is one in a class of antibiotic medications called fluoroquinolones and is produced as a generic or unbranded drug by the name of levofloxacin. These products are prescribed widely to treat bacterial infections and are commonly given for pneumonia, bronchitis, sinusitis, and urinary tract infections. Levaquin was approved by the Food and Drug Administration (FDA) for bacterial infection, but not for virus pathogens. However, it has been widely prescribed almost with abandon, without confirmation that an ailment is bacterial, used off-label (more about that later), and used as a prevention from infection while you are in the hospital or other institution.

Levaquin is commonly prescribed as an oral medication, but can be given intravenously and is found in some eye drops. It became the leading antibiotic sold in this country and resulted in huge profits for its manufacturer for years before becoming available in unbranded generic form.

Another widely used fluoroquinolone in this class is Cipro, or ciprofloxacin as it is known in generic form. It is manufactured by Bayer. Patented in 1980 and introduced in 1987, it is used to treat bacterial infections as well as diseases of the bones and joints, for diarrhea, typhoid fever and respiratory, skin and urinary tract infections as well as other conditions.

Other fluoroquinolones include Avelox (moxifloxacin), Factive (Gemifloxacin), and ofloxacin.[1] You can be sure that if a drug's name ends in floxacin, it is a member of this class of drugs.

These particular antibiotics work by targeting enzymes in the cells of bacteria which stop the cell from replicating its DNA. By not being able to replicate, the bacteria are destroyed. The medicines can be very effective. However, they are able to penetrate tissues throughout the body, including those of the nervous and musculoskeletal system, even crossing the brain barrier to affect functions of the brain. This situation can cause damage to normal tissues as well.[2]

Public Citizen's Health Research Group designates Avelox and Factive as "Do Not Use" drugs. Avelox is reported to be no more effective than other fluoroquinolones but it can cause fatal heart rhythm changes. Factive concerns are about potentially serious skin reactions and heart rhythm changes that could also lead to sudden death. Levaquin, Cipro and ofloxacin are named by this watchdog group as Limited Use drugs.[3] Some of the warnings that are listed on labels or named in research studies include toxic psychosis, muscle damage, seizures, heart arrhythmias, abnormal liver function and kidney damage.[4]

VICTIMS OF THESE drugs insist that they have been "floxed" and refer to themselves as "floxies." The name may sound flippant but the side effects and bodily damages these patients have suffered are serious, even devastating. The term relates to that word floxacin which appears in almost all names of the generics.

Some of the more heartrending stories I encountered include these:

John Fratti suffered for three years with what he called "daily mental and physical damage" from Levaquin. "Every single day," he says, "I have burning nerve pain and tendon issues. In addition, I have a constellation of neurological symptoms. Severe insomnia, tremors, chemical sensitivities, food intolerances, head pressure, vision damage, ataxia, floaters, body shaking, and equilibrium problems."

Prior to taking Levaquin, Fratti said that he was in great health. "I used to play basketball and racquetball. I was very athletic and rarely ever got sick. I led a very clean life. I didn't smoke, didn't drink, didn't do anything illegal. I earned my master's degree as well. I was simply given a legal drug and now my life has been ruined like thousands of others."

Fratti decided to document his experience in an effort to help educate the public about the risks of taking these antibiotics. He established a blog at www.levaquinadversesideeffect.com to tell his story, relate the heartbreaking experiences of others, and provide information about the damage that can be caused by fluoroquinolones. The site is a valuable resource, written by a victim who used to be a sales representative for a pharmaceutical company.

Fratti was one of two fluoroquinolone victims featured on a *PBS Newshour* documentary about the adverse effects of these meds. Featured on that same program was a woman named Jenne Wilcox, a young California schoolteacher, who had been given a one of these drugs prior to sinus surgery to defray any potential post-op infection. The reaction was catastrophic.

"I could barely cope with searing pain from head to toe—on a scale of 1-10 it was relentlessly a 10 plus," she said. For more than a year, she lived in a medical bed in her living room, nearly motionless, depending on round-the-clock care from family.

"Prior to taking this antibiotic," she said, "I was a very healthy, active, happy young woman in my twenties." Afterwards, she became intolerant to caffeine, sugar, MSG, soy, sulfites, aspartame, dairy, gluten, artificial sweeteners, starchy foods high in carbs, nightshade vegetables, and fruits and grains. Eating those foods would cause muscle twitching, itching, nausea, weakness, shaking, stomach upset and more.[5]

One of Oprah's Winfrey's television show producers, Alice McGee, was prescribed a fluoroquinolone for a urinary tract infection. According to Alice, not long after she started taking her pills, she became dizzy, disoriented, began hallucinating and had vivid nightmares. Her vision was so impaired she began bumping into other cars in the parking lot. She saw a long marble staircase in the television studio as a smooth surface, like a long slide. When Alice looked at the drug package insert, she saw that most of the troubles she was having were in the list of side effects. However, she continued to believe that her problems were actually being caused by job-related stress. The executive producer told her to take a day off. Alice mistakenly left her drugs in the office and went without them the next morning at home. By midafternoon, some of the worst symptoms started to go away. It was only then that she realized what was the source of her troubles. In response, Alice did some research, found other individuals who had had adverse reactions to fluoroquinolones and experts who knew about these drugs. They appeared on "Oprah" to share their stories and expertise.[6]

That happened way back in 1993. Early media exposure, little or no impact.

More recently, when presidential candidate Hillary Clinton stumbled and collapsed in 2016 as she approached her car following a political campaign appearance, there was speculation on whether she suffered from exhaustion or some other problem. The media reported that two days before, she had been diagnosed with pneumonia and given an antibiotic called Levaquin, commonly prescribed for that illness.

"It's important to note that Hillary's event that occurred on Sunday could potentially be an adverse reaction with this (fluoroquinolone) drug," Dr. Charles Bennett told *The Daily Caller.* Bennett is a noted oncologist with expertise in medication safety and efficacy.

"You don't know why that event occurred, but it definitely was not normal," he said. Dr. Bennett noted that Levaquin's side effects can include confusion, an inability to walk, weakness and a lack of coordination. Hillary's age at the time placed her in the senior citizen category, an age group that is not recommended for taking this drug unless an illness or condition appears to be severe or life-threatening.[7]

As I continued scouring the internet, it got worse. I came upon more horrific stories. There were endless numbers of people who were suffering and I was overcome by heartrending accounts of injury and pain. Hundreds and hundreds had posted agonizing experiences. Pages of victim photos and their stories appeared on a website called The Fluoroquinolone Wall of Pain (www.fqwallofpain.com). I found postings such these:

I took one dose (500mg) and had SEVERE nightmares, hallucinations, and suicidal thoughts. I'm still dealing with depression and anxiety to this day. I was prescribed for a simple sinus infection! Mark Steirno.

I suffered severe nerve damage and muscle wasting. I had over 30 side effects from taking three doses of Avelox, which is a cousin of Levaquin. Carolyn Spyropoulos.

I have chronic tendonitis, ruptured rotator cuffs, and peripheral neuropathy from being bombarded with moxifloxacin. All the tendons in my body are mush from being pumped full of that drug for years. All my nerve endings burn. Debbie T.

My first big clue that I had a problem was a partially ruptured Achilles heel tendon after a 10-day regime of Cipro. Then horrible back pains, sciatica, damage to the cartilage between disks, ataxia, wobbling [and] stumbling whenever I get excited, joyful, anxious or in unfamiliar places. Brain scan showed nothing. Dee Rohe.

My ten-year-old son has been suffering for the last two years after taking the antibiotic. His eyesight is steadily diminishing because of swelling behind the eyes and damage to his retinas. He is only a child. Please advise. Yvonne Robinson.

I am beside myself. I went to ER for a problem breathing, was diagnosed with bronchitis and treated with levofloxacin, 750 mg and prednisone. By the 5th day in bed I started to have severe pain in my shoulder. By the 6th day it was behind my right knee, so painful & difficult to walk not to mention not being able to get up from a sitting position. I then began to read the paper that you get from the pharmacy and wow this was happening to me…and I was outraged that no one had informed me of what could happen. Geraldine.

What is it like to be severely floxed? You wake up every day in a nightmare that you can't get out of. You wake every day in pain. You become fragile and weak. You injure yourself easily. You feel 100 years old. Your IQ feels like it is dropping by the day. Your body creaks, grinds and pops. You can no longer do any of the things that made life fun and enjoyable. You no longer exercise. You try all day long to find Drs., information on the internet, anything that will help you. You spend countless hours on floxie hope and various Facebook groups trying to find help. You look into candida overgrowth. Fluoride poisoning. Leaky gut. Mercury poisoning. You become obsessed. You become paranoid. You think what other types of evil chemicals has man concocted and are they in my food, water supply etc. You read many studies on fluoroquinolones that don't help you. You cut out gluten. You cut out GMOs. You try various diets. You cut out anything that has antibiotics in it. You eat only organic.

You can no longer go to a restaurant with your wife on a date. You buy books. You read them. They don't help. You take supplements to try to reverse this horrific nightmare. You avoid people because your brain isn't working. You lose friendships. You become isolated. You find yourself crying at work or at random times. You want to do fun things with your family but you can't. You can only watch tv and movies now. You used to be the active dad that played soccer with her daughter and all of the other kids but now you watch. You watch life go by from the sidelines. You want intimacy with your wife but your body doesn't always work like it used to and you don't have the drive you used to. You stop going to church because being social is too stressful for you. You become forgetful. You can't remember things you did earlier in the day. You find yourself falling behind on yard maintenance, things around the house, bills etc. You feel like you are failing your family. Mowing the yard is a workout and painful. You can barely make it through the day at work. You avoid contact with coworkers because you know you aren't right anymore. You become silent. You aren't funny anymore. You don't have a personality anymore. People start to think you are weird, antisocial, lazy but really you just can't think and you hurt all of the time. You want to walk out of work, out of your life but you have bills to pay and a family to provide for. You are anxious. You are beyond stressed out. You pray for healing constantly. Eventually you start to pray for death, for terminal cancer, anything that has an end in sight. Anything that will end this nightmare. Anything that will end the pain… This type of thing shouldn't happen from taking an antibiotic 4.5 years ago but it did. Sadly, it will continue to happen to others. How many people (especially the elderly) are out there going through the same thing but have no clue it was an antibiotic they took years prior?? Andrew.

THE FDA MAINTAINS a site called MedWatch to which patients, physicians and manufacturers are asked to report adverse side effects from taking any drug. Levaquin reports began in 1997 and totaled 21,932 by the end of 2018. They included 668 deaths. Cipro data started coming in in 1983 and added up to another 11,401 reports with an additional 302 deaths. Avelox notifications began in 1997. There were 14,159 complaints posted as well as 571 deaths. Almost all accounts were considered severe or disabling. These 47,492 statistics most likely reflect a small proportion of those harmed by fluoroquinolones. The FDA as well as multiple other sources agree that *only 5 to 10 percent of adverse effects from drugs that happen in the U.S. are reported to the MedWatch site.*[8]

Lawsuits against J&J have increased since an FDA warning advised that Levaquin and other antibiotics in this class had serious risks. Plaintiffs in Pennsylvania and New Jersey, for example, sued J&J claiming that the company marketed Levaquin aggressively even though it knew this powerful antibiotic could cause peripheral neuropathy, a painful nerve condition. Other J&J lawsuits suggest that the company committed fraud by failing to adequately warn doctors and consumers about neuropathy risks earlier. To date, J&J has faced more than 3,400 lawsuits over its drug's links to tendon problems. Many have been settled before going to trial.[9] There has been only one Levaquin lawsuit win. That was back in 2010 in Minnesota and it paid $1.8 million to the plaintiff.[10]

The FDA in 2006 quietly added a new requirement to its regulations. The agency stated that a suing patient must *prove that a company intentionally committed fraud, a corporate crime difficult if not impossible to prove*[11]

The pages of information that are issued with your prescription are required to list adverse events that can occur when you take that drug. One of the most glaring omissions for years was that *fluoroquinolones can cause irreversible damage*. The FDA has since issued a warning about this but it may or may not appear in the flyer. John Fratti believes that handouts given with them should warn that there can *be prolonged, delayed or irreversible central nervous system disorders.*

Not all of the damaging symptoms may be listed in a prescription flyer. The Quinolone Vigilance Foundation (QVF) details these manifestations, which can happen as a single incident or several side effects at the same time.

Peripheral neuropathy
Head pressure
Tinnitus (ringing in the ears)
Rapid heart rate
Tendonitis, tendonosis
Burning sensations in muscles
Inability to walk

Pain
Heel pain
Ruptured Achilles tendons
Insomnia
Nightmares
Brain fog
Joint arthritis
Anxiety
Depression
Ataxia (inability to control muscles)
Chronic fatigue
Headaches
Dry eyes
Difficulty concentrating
Cold hands and feet
Retina damage
And more…

Adverse effects reported to QVF happened to the musculoskeletal, peripheral and central nervous, dermatological, gastrointestinal, vision, ear-nose-and-throat, cardiovascular, endocrine, urinary, reproductive, dental, general constitution, psychological and social systems. In addition, QVF said that there were reports of food or hormonal triggers that might have been caused by these medications.[12] Extreme psychological effects have led to thoughts of suicide.

An article in *Advances in Pharmacological Sciences* suggested that a fluoroquinolone should not be administered during pregnancy, especially in early stage or high doses, to avoid possible fetal defects and abnormalities.[13] A Canadian study revealed that these antibiotics can cause aortic aneurysms and retinal detachments as well as tendon ruptures.[14] Other research has shown that older people on steroids may be more susceptible to tendon tears when taking fluoroquinolones.[15] Children given fluoroquinolone ear drops have been found to be significantly more likely to experience perforated eardrums than those who use an alternative medication.[16]

Scientists recently revealed that there is a link between heart problems and these antibiotics. They found that there was a 2.4 times greater risk of developing aortic and mitral regurgitation, where blood backflows into the heart, when taking Cipro as compared to taking amoxicillin.[17] Taking fluoroquinolones is associated with a more than a twofold increase in the risk of developing aortic aneurysms or aortic tears, although there is still little scientific evidence. Even so, there were 71 cases of aortic aneurysm tears reported to the FDA through April 2018 that had occurred during or after treatment with these medications. The drugs are associated with collagen degradation, which is recognized as a possible cause of tendon rupture. It is that same collagen that is a major component of Achilles tendons and 80 to 90 percent of the aorta.[18]

It seems that some people are devastated by taking only one or two of these pills while others take the entire five or 10-day dosage before experiencing symptoms. Some have had no problems with a previous prescription, but suffer adversely with a later dosage. Some have mild to moderate events. Others become lifelong cripples. Some have recurring problems years after the initial adversity. Many patients take them year after year and have no reactions whatsoever.

VICTIMS REPORT THAT their physicians have few or no recommendations for relief or cure. Often a patient is surfed around from doctor after doctor to try and find a diagnosis, seeking to find a reason for the injurious side effects. Floxies have been told that "once the drug gets out of your system, you will feel better." One patient was told he had been suddenly crippled by a "bad infection." He felt further insulted by being told by board-certified medical professionals that they were "clueless" as to the reason for his symptoms."[19]

Doctors may order a series of tests including bloodwork, MRIs, x-rays, ultrasounds, nerve conduction studies, etc. Reports usually come back negative. One physician suggested taking "an antacid such as Tums to absorb the extra Levaquin still in the system." Another doctor told a patient with neuropathy that it was caused by menopausal hot flashes. Emergency Room personnel called a patient crazy. Patients tell story after story about doctors who emphatically deny that these pills could do such damage.

Dr. Miriam van Staveren went on holiday in 2014 to the Canary Islands and caught an infection. Her ears and sinuses throbbed so she went to see the resort doctor, who prescribed a six-day course of the popular antibiotic levofloxacin. Three weeks later after she got home, her Achilles tendons started to hurt, then her knees and shoulders. She developed shooting pains in her legs and feet, as well as fatigue and depression. "I got sicker and sicker," she said. "I was in pain all day." Previously an active tennis player and hiker, the 61-year-old physician could barely walk, and had to climb the stairs on all fours. She saw a variety of specialists. Some dismissed her symptoms as psychosomatic, others suggested fibro-myalgia or chronic fatigue syndrome. Van Staveren is convinced, however, that it was the antibiotic that poisoned her. In spite of her medical training, van Staveren was unable to find another doctor who believed her. "I want doctors to be informed about the risks, no matter how rare or not they are," she said. "I want warnings all over and I want the warnings to be taken seriously."[20]

If you have a fluoroquinolone reaction, you are pretty much on your own. Ideas for treatment and support can be found in books, newspapers, magazines, television interviews, web sites, blogs, forums and all over the internet, but rarely in the doctor's office.

The renowned Mayo Clinic has produced guidelines for use of fluoroquinolones specifically for athletes, which suggests that this might be a common condition with those who are physically active. The first guideline states: "Athletes should avoid all use of fluoroquinolone antibiotics unless no alternative is available." The advice further states: "Oral or injectable corticosteroids should not be administrated concomitantly with fluoroquinolones."

THERE WAS A well-known research study conducted some years ago about people who died from the adverse effects of their medications. It concluded that an estimated 106,000 Americans succumbed from adverse events after taking their medicines. Researchers only studied hospitalized patients, not additional deaths outside of the hospital such as in nursing homes, retirement facilities or at home. [21]

Reporting of such deaths is sketchy. Death certificates, according to a director of forensic operations at an Iowa morgue, most likely would record a patient's demise from adverse medical effects as a "natural" death or as the disease the patient had been treated for rather than death caused by meds.[22]

It's difficult to come up with an exact number of injuries from taking medicines. Doctors are reluctant to admit that they might have caused patient harm. They may fear lawsuits or patients making reports to associations that have accredited them. Or, they may not want their patients to lose confidence in their professional abilities. Patient reporting to medical associations is complicated and rarely done.

The National Institutes of Health concludes that symptoms may suddenly occur months or years after an initial adverse reaction and may persist with no treatment being effective.[23] These situations add to the difficulty of detecting how many fluoroquinolone injuries have actually occurred.

THE FIRST FLOXED individual to suggest scientifically that fluoroquinolones can cause irreversible damage to the DNA (the genetics that make up your individualized cell structure) was Joe King, PhD, a mathematician and professor at Carnegie Mellon Research University, a consultant to corporations worldwide, a competitive body builder and a concert pianist. Here is his abbreviated story:

On New Year's Eve 2009, my father and I went to a local restaurant to have dinner. Two hours after eating a meal of grilled chicken, I was in the ER bent over with excruciating abdominal pain, chills, and a severe headache. I was diagnosed with salmonella food poisoning.

The ER doctor started an IV infusion of 750 mg of Levaquin. Within thirty minutes I went into convulsions. The doctor blamed it on the salmonella. I then received Levaquin 1,000 mg a day orally for a total of twenty-eight days, then Cipro for another seven days. With each day, I became progressively more incapacitated. I was in and out of the hospital three to four times per week. The third week I was also given prednisone for the excruciating muscle and tendon pain.

On the third day of this regimen, my Achilles tendon and other tendons began rupturing while I was trying to sleep. Both tendons ruptured seven months later, while I was simply watching television.

Two years later, I was hospitalized for long periods while my doctors searched for answers. All during this time, not one doctor attributed my declining health to fluoroquinolones. Meanwhile, it was strongly suggested to me that my health complaints were psychosomatic. By the end of 2011, I had lost eighty pounds and my muscle mass had dropped, continued deterioration of the nerves in my heart and other areas left me with continuous pain.

In 2012, I developed a collapsed coronary artery, which is frequently fatal, while at the vet's office with my cat. I went into cardiac shock. The hospital sent me home and suggested I call hospice. My friends came to the hospital to carry me home to die.

I saw an attorney's ad on television asking people if they'd had tendon ruptures, muscle pain, heart problems, etc. Immediately I contacted him and, finally, for the first time, someone explained why I became so sick and incapacitated. I contacted the toxicologist at the Dade County Medical Examiner's Office and asked if he could run a DNA test for me. He directed me to an FBA-certified toxicology lab [where my] DNA was analyzed by the most modern methods [and the researcher] informed me that fluoroquinolones and some metabolites were found attached abnormally to my DNA. Next, she contacted some heavyweights in the fields of pharmaceutical toxicology, research and development. She also contacted several medical schools and research facilities across the country, including the Utah School of Medicine's Center for Human Poisoning. Thus, we involved the very top toxicology resources anywhere. The unanimous conclusion was that my DNA had been [changed] by Levaquin and Cipro. This was the first conclusive proof in the world that fluoroquinolones truly damaged human DNA.

The experts also had another message for me: the effect of the fluoroquinolone poisoning was irreversible. Several weeks later, I collapsed in my backyard and was taken to the same ER. The doctors immediately

[said], "Why are you back? We told you there is nothing wrong with you." I threw my toxicology report at them. They read the report [and] immediately changed the way they dealt with me. I no longer had doubtful doctors who were dismissive, sometimes insulting [such as saying] "Mr. King, there is nothing wrong with you! Do not come back to this ER and tie it up when we have real sick people waiting to get help!"

Dr. King has been spreading the word relentlessly about the potential dangers of these medicines. He testified in a wheelchair at a Senate committee hearing and recommended that the FDA be pressured to initiate studies to investigate fluroquinolones and provide actions that should be taken.

AMERICANS LIVE IN a pill culture. Prescription medicines are the rule of thumb when you're sick or injured. We are quite literally overdosed on pills. Many are prescribed like water, like candy, to make us feel better, to meet our demands for meds, to fight minimal infection and slight pain. Older people ingest more pills than any other age group, some of which are unnecessary or have risk of interactions with the many other meds they are taking.

Overuse by the elderly is common. Nearly half of Americans age sixty-five and older take five or more drugs or supplements every week. Twelve percent take 10 or more prescriptions. Government studies found that almost 18% of all Medicare patients were taking meds that were not safe for older people. Elderly are said to be more susceptible to manipulation by drug company advertising and ask their doctors for those pills. Doctors sometimes add a new antidote on top of old ones when new symptoms appear. What if the new symptoms are just a side effect of the medication they are currently taking?[24]

We are an enormously overprescribed populace that especially affects those of advanced age. According to Dr. Arnold Relman, professor emeritus at Harvard Medical School, seniors over and over again are getting far more pills than they need. "The average senior in America is probably taking twice or three times the medications they require," he says.[25]

Dentists are the fourth most frequent prescribers of oral antibiotics in the U.S., accounting for one in ten pharmacy prescriptions. Many are taken before procedures in the belief that they will prevent infection from the release of bacteria from the mouth into the bloodstream. It has been suggested that more than three-quarters of these treatments are unnecessary.[26]

The downside to antibiotic overuse is that we are becoming resistant to these drugs. They are not working as efficiently if at all. Programs have been initiated worldwide to educate the medical establishment about the dangers of overuse. The World Congress on Antibiotics estimates that drug-resistant bacteria infect at least 2 million Americans each year and kill 23,000. An analysis commissioned by the United Kingdom's prime minister and the Wellcome Trust predicted that drug-resistant infections could kill 10 million people a year worldwide by 2050.[27]

IN 2016, THE specter of Ciprofloxacin being used as a herbicide was discussed by scientists in Australia, who discovered that this antibiotic appeared to be effective for killing weeds. According to Dr. Josh Mylne at the University of Western Australia, "it kills plants in a very similar fashion to the way it kills microbes, by binding and interfering with an enzyme called gyrase." If Cipro comes to be used as a spray on crops to kill weeds, it would make its way into the food system, cause harm to humans, and increase antibiotic resistance.[28]

In December 2017 oral, intravenous and optic Levaquin were quietly taken off the market by their maker. According to Dr. Charles Bennett, "Levaquin was only about 1% of the market share and 99% was generic. It was hard for them to make money given the lawsuits they were facing."[29]

Brand names including Cipro, Avelox, Factive, and Baxdela as well as Levaquin have more than 60 generic equivalents which are currently being sold to the public worldwide. Because generics are exact copies of the original drugs, they all have the same serious risks.[30]

This class of drugs can and does do irreparable harm. When prescribed appropriately, however, these medicines can save lives that would not have been saved by other means.

WHAT TO DO

- If you develop severe pain or highly abnormal symptoms after taking ANY prescription medication, call your doctor immediately. Do not wait. Call 911 if your doctor is unavailable.

- If you are a victim of a fluoroquinolone adverse reaction, you may want to join the many online discussion and support groups that are available. *(See Resources Section.)*

- Become informed about your medications. Read the prescription flyers that come with them. Heed their warnings.

- You have a right to question your doctor or hospital staff about the pills that are going into your body. You have a right to receive answers and not to be brushed off or belittled.

- Don't take an antibiotic unless it is necessary. In the case of Levaquin or Cipro, for example, it is suggested that they are to be used in serious medical situations or life-threatening illness only.

- Eat animal products that are labeled "raised without antibiotics" and organics that are "grown without antibiotics."

- Ask your caregiver about possible interactions with other medications you are taking. Do not take fluoroquinolones with steroids, such as cortisone, during or after any adverse reaction.

- There are numerous treatment suggestions floating around the Internet. Some are radical. Be careful. Consult with a certified professional before trying new therapies, over-the-counter drugs, or dietary supplements.

- Become informed about what fluoroquinolones are and their potential side effects. Become an advocate for safe prescribing. It's okay to discuss these issues with your doctor. Talk to your friends, your family, and your caregivers about the possible harm that can occur from taking these drugs.

HOW DID WE get into this situation where there are life-saving drugs such as these that cause so many harmful side effects? How did they come to be? How did these powerful medications become so frequently prescribed worldwide even though they are causing serious physical and mental damage? To answer these questions, one needs to understand what goes on in the pharmaceuticals industry, which has grown to become so enormous it is known as Big Pharma.

Notes

1   "FDA Requires Stronger Warnings for Commonly Used Antibiotics." *Worst Pills Best Pills Newsletter*, February 2017.

2   Monti, Adrian. "Common antibiotics doctors say could give you organ failure as millions of Britons are at risk of devastating permanent side effects as a result of over-prescribing." *Daily Mail*, October 27, 2018.

3   "FDA Requires Stronger Warnings for Commonly Used Antibiotics." *Worst Pills Best Pills Newsletter*, February 2017.

4   Haiken, Melanie. "Antibiotic Alert: The Drug the Doctor Ordered Could Cause Deadly Side Effects." www.forbes.com, September 20, 2012.

5   "The Road to Recovery After a Side Effect Changed One Woman's Life." www.news.goraw.com, March, 2014.

6   Fried, Stephen. *Bitter Pills, Inside the Hazardous World of Legal Drugs*, Bantam Books, New York, NY, 1999, pp. 114-115.

7   "Hillary Clinton and Levaquin, A Teachable Moment." www.myquinstory.info, September 16, 2016.

8   www.fda.gov.

9   Staton, Tracy. "A new wave of Levaquin lawsuits, patients claim J&J knew about nerve-damage risks." *FiercePharma*,

10 "Consumer Wins Levaquin Lawsuit." www.aboutlawsuits.com, December 10, 2010.

11 Gotzsche, Peter C. *Deadly Medicines and Organised Crime.* Radcliffe Publishing Ltd., London, 2013, p.111.

12 www.saferpills.org. Quinolone Vigilance Foundation.

13 Aboubakr, Mohamed et al. "…administration of norfloxacin during pregnancy. Advances in Pharmacological Sciences, February 3, 2014.

14 Daneman, Nick et al. "Fluoroquinolones and collagen-associated severe adverse events: a longitudinal cohort study." *CIDRAP News*, November 18, 2015.

15 Park, Alice. "A Cautionary Tale About Antibiotics." *Time Magazine*, April 14, 2017.

16 Airwisan, Adel, et al. "Study Shows that Quinolone Ear Drops Increase Rates of Eardrum Perforation in Children." www.floxiehope.com, April 24, 2017.

17 *NCI Well Connect*, Dec 2, 2019.

18 www.DrugWatch.com, January 22, 2020.

19 www.floxiehope.com. "B's Recovery Story—Levaquin Toxicity."

20 Marchant, Jo. "When antibiotics turn toxic." *Nature*, March 21, 2018.

21 Petersen, Melody. *Our Daily Meds*, Picador, New York, NY, 2008, p. 304.

22 Ibid, p. 305.

23 Michalak, K. et al. "Treatment of the Fluoroquinolone-Associated Disability: The Pathobiochemical Implications." www.ncbi.nim.nih.gov, Epub, September 2017.

24 Petersen, Melody. *Our Daily Meds*, pp. 299-301.

25 Ibid, p. 7.

26 AbulDagga, Azza, MHA, PhD. "Most Preventive Antibiotics Before Dental Procedures Are Unnecessary, Study Finds." *Health Letter*, December 2019.

27 "Drug-resistant bacteria infect at least 2 million…" Posted by Kathleen D'Souza, ANTIBIOTIC DAMAGE!, www.facebook.com, May 15, 2018. Stats from the World Congress on Antibiotics.

28 Dessy, Mira. "Antibiotic Weedkiller." *The Ingredient Guru*, www.theingredientguru.com, November, 2016.

29 "Drug maker stopped making popular antibiotic Levaquin amid concerns about mental health side effects." RTV6, Tampa Bay, FL, July 17, 2018.

30 Cox, Emily. "Levaquin Pulled from Market to Avoid FDA Action." Arentz Law Group, July 22, 2018.

THE INFLUENCE OF BIG PHARMA

*As the pharmaceutical industry has
devoted itself to aggressive promotion,
it has been transformed from one with
the ability to do great good to one that
is causing far too much needless harm.*

MELODY PETERSEN, *OUR DAILY MEDS*

BIG PHARMA, THE group of gigantic companies that make up most of the pharmaceutical industry, produces almost all medicinal drugs sold in the United States. The industry sells billions of dollars of drugs each year. Americans take more pills than any other other country. Between 2010 and 2017, pill consumption rose 85% compared to a population that went up by only 21%.

Too many medicines are unneeded, are taken prematurely, for too long a time, or may have adverse interactions. Popping pills has become a bad habit in America with some very serious consequences.

Most of us take a prescription drug of some kind. We swallow four pharmaceuticals on average and many of us also take over-the-counter (OTC) drugs as well as vitamins and mineral supplements. Consumption has tripled in the last 20 years. With that, there has been a parallel rise in harm from unnecessary prescription use, dangerous drug interactions, and questionable supplements.

Seniors consume even more prescriptions: 40 percent take five or more prescribed drugs. Older people often are more at risk of harm from drugs because of their age and the mix of medicines they take.

Nearly 1.3 million people went to an emergency room in 2014 due to an adverse effect from a drug and 124,000 died, according to data from the FDA and Centers for Disease Control and Prevention (CDC). Still, 73% of Americans say they are not all that concerned about a drug's side effects.[1]

HOW POWERFUL ANTIBIOTICS such as fluoroquinolones got here is a story that began with medical discoveries and remedies provided by a caring and ethical pharmaceutical industry, but has since grown to become a huge business that focuses on profits. The new narrative includes widespread deception, greed and manipulation.

It was not always so. The president of pharmaceutical giant Merck in December 1950 said: "We try never to forget that medicine is for the people. It is not for the profits. The profits follow." Merck had just commercially produced cortisone, a drug that helped crippled and bedridden people not only to walk again, but to climb stairs and even dance.

Some years before that, when penicillin was discovered quite by accident in England, Merck initially refused to be involved in its manufacture, even though this first antibiotic was a sure cure for pneumonia and bacterial infections and was desperately needed to treat WWII troops. Penicillin was not easy to produce in quantity. Merck said it didn't want to spend time trying to find out how to mass produce this new life-saving drug. Fortunately, the company was convinced to change its mind. This greatest drug discovery of all time up until then was thankfully being mass-produced by Merck by the time D-Day rolled around.[2]

At one time medicines to treat human frailties, illness and disease used to be home remedies or antidotes passed down from generation to generation. Plants had always been a source of relief or healing.

However, in the 1800s and early 1900s patent medicine took hold. Quacks discovered that anyone could produce nostrums, syrups, and elixirs without testing, concoct them from any ingredient, and sell them anywhere and everywhere. And they did. There were hundreds of patent medicine frauds, tonics that promised cures but often delivered dangerous drugs or simply alcohol, morphine or even cocaine to make you "feel better" or "cure what ails you."

Who could resist ads touting "Hale's Honey of Horehound & Tar for the speedy cure of coughs, colds, influenza, sore throats, lung and all bronchial complaints" or "Paine's Celery Compound" for nervousness and insomnia? A gullible public ate it up.

One Chicago physician claimed that the patent medicine industry was the most gigantic swindle ever perpetrated on the American public. Sales zoomed upwards with a boost from advertising, a lesson noted by the pharmaceutical industry later on and used effectively to sell billions of prescription drugs.

In 1930, the FDA began to curb sales of those tonics, but it wasn't until a legally marketed antidote called Elixir of Sulfanilamide led to 107 deaths in 1937 that legislation finally closed most of the remaining legal loopholes for patent medicine.[3]

Merck in that same year sold primarily natural botanicals or chemicals such as digitalis, aspirin, morphine and insulin. They were sold without prescription. But then drug companies saw that there was a need to treat conditions caused by people living longer—heart disease, cancer and stroke—which required more complicated compounds.

Industry began to believe that scientific standards set by a government agency such as an FDA could drive a great engine of discovery and sales. Pharmaceutical companies would create brand new drugs and get approval by meeting standards set by an agency outside the industry. They would require that those medicines be sold by prescription only with prices set by each company.[4]

A new day was born, and a dark side developed. Providing simple medicines to do great good morphed into new lab-created medications that could cause needless harm. Fluoroquinolones could be the poster child.

IT WAS IN the 1960s that fluorine atoms were added to antibiotics called quinolones and they became fluoroquinolones. Adding this allowed the new antibiotics to penetrate tissues throughout the body, including the central nervous system, and boosted their effectiveness against a broad range of bacterial infections.[5]

The fluoroquinolone ciprofloxacin (Cipro) was patented by Bayer in 1980 and introduced in 1987. The fluoroquinolone development program at Bayer focused on examining the effects of minor changes to the structure of norfloxacin. Bayer added one carbon atom to that drug resulting in a two to 10-fold increase in potency against Gram-negative bacteria, germs which cause pneumonia and meningitis and blood stream, wound or surgical site infections.

Ciprofloxacin is on the World Health Organization's List of Essential Medicines, a compilation of the most effective and safe medicines needed in a health system. It is available as a generic medication and not very expensive. The wholesale cost in the developing world is between three cents and 13 cents per pill. In the U.S. it is sold for about 40 cents per dose. In 2016, seven million prescriptions were sold.

Ciprofloxacin is the most widely-used of the second-generation of fluoroquinolones. Back in 2010, more than 20 million prescriptions were written, making it the fifth most commonly prescribed drug in the U.S. and the 35th most-prescribed generic drug.

As for the development of levofloxacin (Levaquin), it was patented in 1985 and approved for medical use in the U.S. in 1996 by J&J in cooperation with its maker, Daichi of Japan. It was approved for treating bacterial sinusitis, bacterial exacerbations of bronchitis, community-acquired pneumonia, uncomplicated skin infections, complicated urinary tract infections, and acute pyelonephritis.

It is also on the World Health Organization's List of Essential Medicines and was approved as a generic in 2009. The wholesale cost of this drug in the developing world is about 44 to 95 cents per one week of treatment. In the U.S. a treatment week costs patients about $50 to $100.

By 1993, levofloxacin had reached blockbuster status. Combined worldwide sales of levofloxacin and ofloxacin, a more potent and toxic formula, had generated $1.6 billion in income for J&J.[6] Predictions are that the fluoroquinolone market will have unusually strong growth by the end of 2025 due to effectiveness against an increasing prevalence of infectious diseases worldwide and resistance to other less powerful antibiotics.[7]

HERE'S HOW THE drug development and approval process proceeds. Pharmaceutical companies do research for new drugs. They spend years and enormous amounts of money, they say, researching and creating these medications. Development includes scientific laboratory work, then clinical trials to determine each drug's effectiveness, then filling out applications to the FDA to gain each drug's approval. Upon approval, the companies are finally able to promote and sell their new product. A long process, but it's even more complicated than that.

Take research. Yes, company scientists do spend time in laboratories looking for new medicines and cures. Drug companies use this argument to justify high drug prices (billions of dollars spent on research and development). But what's the real story about this "make-believe billion," as writer Timothy Noah calls it?

He wrote that an average of *$2.6 billion* in research and development was reportedly spent per company to develop each new drug. This figure was the result of a 2016 survey conducted by the Tufts Center for the Study of Drug Development; an organization funded by the drug companies themselves. The conclusion was based upon unverified data submitted by only 10 of 24 pharmaceutical companies.[8] Similar research by Tufts five years before had set the figure at a lower $1.2 billion. This revealed a questionable and unexplained dramatic rise of $1.4 billion in research and development costs that somehow doubled in only five years.[9]

Noah found that very little of a new drug's costs for the first research phase, the lab part, is funded by industry. Almost 85% is paid for and conducted by government groups. Private universities also fund drug research and development. On top of this, Big Pharma gets a huge 39% research tax break on profits, not depreciated over time like other investments.

Noah wrote that noted sociologist Donald W. Light and economist Rebecca Warburton analyzed the Tufts research. They came up with $59 million in actual research costs per company, *$2.1 billion less than reported in the industry-supported study.*[10]

Of course, not all drugs under development make it to the marketplace. How many are under development is not public information. Industry says this information should remain secret because competition could profit by it. Pharmaceutical executives say that

95% of experimental drugs fail. Medicine development expert Susan Desmond-Hellman read this and said: "This is crazy. Any businessperson would look at this and say, 'You can't make a business of this. This is not a good investment.'"[11]

Many public government agencies such as the National Institutes of Health (NIH) fund research projects for drug companies with taxpayers covering the costs. Public Citizen reported that of 26 innovative and groundbreaking drugs or classes of them that were approved by the FDA between 1984 and 2009, only a minority were developed exclusively within industry.

Instead of inventing a medicine, companies may buy smaller companies that have already developed a drug, perhaps with federal funds. They might recoup the purchase price during the first or second year of sales by employing high-powered marketing. Big company mergers in recent years bring cost advantages as well as the ability to secure drugs already developed. Those older drugs can be re-marketed with dramatically-increased prices, especially if there is no longer any competition for them.[12]

A trend in recent years is for companies to develop what are called "orphan drugs," medications for rare diseases. Once developed, they can sell them to the smaller markets as life-saving or curative pills at incredibly-inflated prices, usually in the hundreds of thousands of dollars per treatment. This happens even as development costs are less than usual due to smaller clinical trials. Fewer rare-diseased patients are available for trials. A federal tax credit for developing exclusive drugs also lowers costs.[13]

Then there are the "Me-Too" pills. These are re-jiggered drugs that include minor changes, are given new names, don't require new FDA clearance, and are marketed with a massive advertising campaign as the latest innovative breakthrough, according to Rosanne Spector, editor of *Stanford Medicine.*[14]

Another practice is for companies to stop discovery research in areas that aren't showing promising profits. Forest Labs, Inc. cut 500 jobs in 2013 in a move to focus efforts on "drug development, not drug discovery." Today's hot industry markets are heart, cancer and stroke as well as rare diseases.

As for new antibiotic drug development, it has slowed markedly. The few antibiotics introduced in this century are basically variations on past themes. Most drug makers have pulled out of the race entirely, eliminating antibiotic research and development in favor of more lucrative medicines.[15] Fluoroquinolones, for example, have been working well for years and selling extremely well. There is no incentive to invent a replacement. Older antibiotics now sold as generics are cheap and in good supply. In addition, because of the huge numbers of patients taking antibiotics, it would be almost impossible to find non-users for clinical trials.[16]

CLINICAL TRIALS ARE the second step in pill development after research determines that a new drug has been created. These trials should be based upon what is called evidence-based medicine. Evidence-based medicine means making conclusions and decisions based upon scientific evidence, truth not bias.

Clinical trials are studies in which animals or humans are tested by one group taking the newly-created medicine and one group taking a placebo, a harmless pill with no health effect. The results show whether the new medicine is effective and whether there are adverse events. All new drugs must pass trials that show effectiveness and small chance of harm.

It is mandated by the FDA that four separate trials for each drug be conducted. Phase 1 tests safety in humans. Phase 2 tests efficacy. Phase 3 confirms safety and efficacy. Phase 4 involves conducting safety studies during the initial sales period.

Hundreds, even thousands, of participants are needed to produce evidence-based results. Participants are recruited and testing begins. Results can be marred by participants dropping out or recruitment being biased or manipulated. Old people who might have more adverse effects than younger participants can be eliminated. Using exclusively all men or all women for a trial could tilt results.

In order to secure positive outcomes, companies sometimes test new drugs with lower doses than a competitor's similar drug, thus skewing results in their favor. They can select specific populations, such as blacks or prisoners or the homeless, most of whom have sketchy records of current or past diseases or allergies that might affect results.

Bad practices, according to Donald Light in his book *The Risks of Prescription Drugs*, include conducting trials that:

- exclude patients who are older, poorer, minority or female because they are more likely to suffer adverse effects

- are short-timed so that they show effectiveness but not toxic side effects that might be revealed later

- are too small to pick up any but the most apparent short-term toxic effects

- record only selected toxic side effects rather than all of them

- rule out patients with other health problems or risks, even if they are likely to be prescribed the drug once approved

- use a comparator drug (if there is one) that has similar adverse effects so that the tested drug's risks don't stand out as statistically significant

- exclude subjects who couldn't tolerate side effects or larger doses

- split adverse effects into subgroups of one or two patients so that they won't be detected statistically

- selectively publish evidence to support marketing[17]

Companies don't have to publicly publish trial data. If they choose not to, it leaves the general public, pharmacists, physicians, patients and caregivers bereft of a medicine's actual trial outcomes and discovered risks.

For 20 years the U.S. government urged any company or institution that conducts clinical trials to record results in a federal database called ClinicalTrials.gov so that doctors and patients can see whether new treatments are safe and effective. Few have consistently done so, even after a 2007 law made posting mandatory. In 2017 the NIH and the FDA tried again. They enacted what they called a "final rule" to clarify the law's expectations and penalties for failing to disclose trial results or register within a deadline. The law took effect in 2018. Two years later, *Science* magazine revealed that many still ignored the requirement and federal officials did little or nothing to enforce the law.

Trials Tracker conservatively estimated that the FDA could have collected more than $6 billion in penalties for trial reports that were overdue or not registered. The agency has yet to demand a single dollar despite more than 2,600 trials that were not filed or were late. The NIH has not withheld a single grant for not posting.

"Public-facing websites run by the government should be accurate. That's not asking much," says Senator Chuck Grassley (R-IA), who advocated for the 2007 law. "It's a question of basic management and agency competence. The government has a duty to police its work product, especially because the public trusts that .gov websites will be accurate and reliable."

Big Pharma has a better record of compliance than universities and medical centers. Institutions such as Harvard University-affiliated Boston Children's Hospital, the MD Anderson Cancer Center and the Mayo Clinic are among those who delayed or avoided required registration of trial results at ClinicalTrials.gov. The consequences of not sharing results is that doctors, researchers and potential trial participants who rely on the site for up-to-date information won't know until later whether new medicines are harmful or ineffective. They will not be apprised of major adverse events that occurred in trials or if there was failure to improve effectiveness beyond other current medications.[18]

INDUSTRY MUST PROVIDE extensive data about clinical trials to the FDA upon seeking drug approval. Data submitted, however, usually highlights the positive results and minimizes those results that might lead to non-approval.

Every year the FDA conducts inspections of several hundred clinical trial sites. During one such inspection detailed in *Internal Medicine*, Charles Seife, MS, discovered that 57 trials showed evidence of one or more of the following:

- falsification of submitted information (39%)

- problems with adverse events reporting (25%)

- protocol violations (74%)

- inadequate recordkeeping (61%)

- failure to protect the safety of patients and/or issues with oversight or informed consent (53%)

- other violations not categorized (35%)

There were no corrections, retractions, expressions of concern or comments acknowledging the key issues identified at this inspection by any of the companies that conducted these clinical studies. And even though fraudulent data were discovered in the inspections, only three of 78 publications that wrote about these trials mentioned the objectionable conditions or practices uncovered by the FDA.[19]

If adverse events are not found in clinical trials or go unreported and the drugs are still approved for sale, the patient becomes the guinea pig. The medications are tested by the general population for benefits and harms. Numerous adverse events, such as have been reported with fluoroquinolones, may be the result of such industry manipulation.

ONCE A DRUG is approved by the FDA, a company gets an exclusive right to market it for a minimum of five to seven years. Most are protected by patents that last 20 years. The reasoning behind patents, which provide the company exclusive promotion and sales of a drug for a period of years, is that the company needs many years of sales at their own set price in order to recover costs and make a profit.

When patents expire, other companies can produce the drug as a generic, which are pills with the same ingredients but that sell for less.

To delay generic manufacture, however, drug companies have been known to secretly make payments to generic drug makers to drop patent challenges and refrain from manufacturing a product. This gives the brand-name company a chance to continue to produce the original drugs for a longer period and continue charging high prices. The Federal Trade Commission (FTC) brought a suit against Endo in Malvern, Pa. alleging that the company violated federal antitrust laws when it was found to be engaging in that practice. Fines were paid. The practice continues.

Another questionable scheme is called "evergreening," whereby a company claims minimal changes in its product so that patents can be re-established and continue beyond the end of the patent period. This practice blocks generics from getting drugs into production.[20]

AFTER A DRUG is approved, the company sets in motion its huge marketing budget. Promotion may even start before approval to garner enthusiasm from the public with the hope of influencing a positive FDA outcome. Marketing efforts include massive television advertising and a heavy push to sell a new drug to physicians. It also includes announcing a new drug in medical journals, creating councils or organizations to promote the pills as well as provide credibility, initiating conferences for physicians and opinion makers to talk up the new medication … and much, much more.

Companies will ask established medical groups to promote new products. They will set up and fund new organizations that sound credible to hype their pills. The public is often unaware that some associations that claim to advocate for patients are heavily funded and influenced by industry. *DrugWatch* recommends that such arrangements be made public so that patients themselves can decide if there is a conflict of interest.[21]

Melody Petersen in her book *Our Daily Meds* interviewed pharmaceutical executives who talked about their company's medicines as if they were Hollywood producers about to release a new film. They spoke of "launching their next blockbuster," which they defined as a medicine that could bring in sales of one billion dollars or more in a single year. Some of their new drugs, she noted, were merely combinations of old drugs or were little different than those already being sold. They simply got a new name and a fresh marketing campaign.

Drug advertising and promotion mirrors what Coca Cola or Proctor and Gamble does. Pharmaceutical ads can be found on billboards, scoreboards, hoods of race cars, on back covers of magazines, and on internet sites. There are coupons, free gifts, sweepstakes, scholarship contests, sponsorships of concerts and golf tournaments and museum exhibitions, videos, and educational events. Other tactics may be creation of national days that celebrate a disease that is successfully treated, surprise, by a company's new pill. Opinion pieces are created for newspapers and news sites to support political and sales efforts. Celebrities are hired as spokespeople and appear in advertising.

Physicians and medical experts are brought on board to lead conferences or seminars. They, as well as celebrities, are featured in ads hyping medical products.

Other subtle and not-so-subtle marketing techniques include promoting drugs at large gatherings such as state fairs or at community healthcare meetings or internet conferences. Marketers reach out through facebook.com pages, write opinion pieces for newspapers that support industry agendas, produce articles for professional medical journals that are ghost-written, i.e. they hide the source by paying professional writers to write them. They also organize professional groups to lobby for them.

Pharmaceutical industry lobby spending in Washington, DC was $78 million in only the first quarter of 2017. This was an increase of 14% over the previous year's first quarter and represented by far the most spent by any lobby group to influence congressional decision-makers.[22] By the end of that year, spending had hit *$300 million and 1,480 lobbyists were representing pharmaceutical interests.*[23]

Drug companies are traditionally among the biggest spenders on political candidates. Twenty of them in 2017 through January of 2018 doled out thousands of dollars to political candidates. Vertex Pharmaceuticals gifted $79,349 to individuals running for seats in the House and Senate, for example, and Merck & Co. donated $458,547.[24]

Big Pharma sometimes pays patients who have successfully used their drugs to promote them in social media. These social media influencers are often trusted more than celebrities when they post ads or positive comments about products and help drive sales. Incidentally, the FDA does not place any restrictions on who can become an influencer. Anyone can be a spokesperson and promote a prescription product.[25]

Detergents and drugs are now promoted in the same way. Television is full of ads for medicines. If it didn't work, they wouldn't be there. Money reportedly spent by Big Pharma across all media was tagged in 2017 at $5.8 billion a year.[26] More recently, researchers estimated that medical marketing has soared to $30 billion, almost double from 20 years ago. Big Pharma ads appeared *five million times in just one year* on TV, in newspapers and magazines, on online sites and elsewhere.[27]

One of the experts who did that research said that this upward trend is concerning and suggested that consumers need to be increasingly skeptical about marketing claims. Of all countries worldwide, only the U.S. and New Zealand allow prescription drugs to be advertised directly to consumers.

Marketing to doctors, nurses and other health professionals has been estimated at $20 billion, spending that includes free drug samples and in-person sales pitches from drug representatives. Spending to promote meds to hospitals or other institutions is in addition to that.

Promotional activities of drug manufacturers have created a demand greater than the actual needs, states the World Health Organization.[28] Doris Burtscher, a medical anthropologist, believes that heavy promotion by pharmaceutical companies has ensured that much of the public has become convinced that there must be a pill for every ill.[29]

As for regulation, federal law says medical advertising must be truthful, not deceptive, and backed by scientific evidence. The FDA oversees prescription drug and medical device ads. The Federal Trade Commission regulates OTC products. There were more than 100,000 submissions to these agencies just in 2016. Analysis suggests that the uncontrolled surge in medical marketing has led to spotty oversight by both agencies. Off-label or deceptive marketing practices have resulted in $11 billion in fines and 103 settlements between drug companies and regulators since 1997.

In 2015, the American Medical Association supported banning direct-to-consumer ads for prescription drugs and said doctors should not accept medical industry payments or gifts intended to influence prescribing habits. The leading industry trade group, Pharmaceutical Research and Manufacturers of America (PhRMA), defended marketing practices and said direct-to-consumer ads can make patients better informed about their health and treatment options. A spokeswoman said these ads also increase awareness of the benefits and risks of new medicines and encourage appropriate use.

An editorial in the *Journal of the American Medical Association (JAMA)* defended medical marketing saying it needs no apologist. It has helped make patients more informed as consumers, the editorial states, and it's up to doctors to help their patients understand product claims. The editors added, however: "Some physicians may need to become educated about deceptive marketing."

Too often, companies entice consumers into purchasing medical products based on deceptive advertisements that overstate the potential benefits of the products and omit key information about risks, writes Dr. Michael Carome in Public Citizen's *Health Letter*.[30] An investigation of 168 ads promoting prescription and OTC drugs showed that 33% were true, based upon available evidence, 57% were potentially misleading, and 10% were outright false. In other words, *two-thirds of the advertising claims were not entirely true or accurate.*[31]

The FDA recently considered whether to give a break to Big Pharma advertising, allowing companies to reduce announcing a long list of side effects now required in drug ads. The agency said that a briefer risk statement in drug ads may improve a viewer's retention of risk information and could promote a better understanding of benefit information. Advertising would have to be accompanied by a disclosure statement that not all risk information was being presented.[32] "Just like the old song," says Dr. Sidney Wolfe of Public Citizen, "the drug companies will get to accentuate the positive and eliminate the negative."[33]

ONE OF THE most egregious promotional tactics by Big Pharma is called "disease mongering." It occurs when a company turns a common or normal medical condition, such as the urge to pee, into a disease, calling it overactive bladder. Miraculously, it can be cured by the company's latest product. It was fibromyalgia for Pfizer and pink Viagra for women. There are medications for conditions called pre-obesity, chemical imbalance, schoolroom restlessness, sadness, even fear of speaking in public. Osteopenia, erectile disfunction, and pediatric bipolar disorder appeared out of nowhere.[34]

A "binge-eating" awareness campaign by one pharmaceutical company took an already known eating condition and created glossy ads about people with this disorder pleading for help. The company running these ads didn't have to advertise their medicine which would combat this behavior. It produced the only drug approved for "overeating disease." Experts say that eating behavior and its associated guilty feelings can be successfully treated through behavioral therapy instead of by pills.[35]

The proliferation of "pre-disease" diagnosis, such as mild bone loss (osteopenia), slightly elevated blood pressure (prehypertension) or pre-diabetes (slightly elevated but still normal blood glucose reading) may be helpful in catching something early before it gets out of hand. However, in far too many cases these pre-disease diagnoses, promoted by pharmaceutical companies, result in prescribing drugs before they are needed. It is Big Pharma that invents and promotes these pre-diseases. Drug companies have, of course, the perfect pill to combat each one of them.[36]

No private industry is held in lower esteem by Americans than the pharmaceutical industry, according to a Gallup poll. Seventy-seven percent of

Americans believe that drug companies are unfairly profiting from lifesaving drugs.

The Pharmaceutical Research and Marketing Association (PhRMA), an industry trade association, launched a multi-million-dollar, multi-year public relations campaign in 2017. Its focus was to promote the overall benefits of the industry and to combat mounting anger at the high costs of drugs, extreme profits, and at increasing criticism of industry tactics.[37]

Pharmaceutical companies are creating a staff position at the senior level called chief design officer. These individuals advise on how to design appealing products, packaging and sales programs to meet today's more informed and increasingly negative market.

"Consumers are much savvier about marketing. What they react to well is cleverly designed products," says Mark Curtis, an executive at a design consultancy that works with health care companies.[38]

PHYSICIANS HAVE BEEN a major target for medicine promotion, including risky fluoroquinolones. Doctors are the final link in the chain to medicate the consumer with company products. Big Pharma spends big to reach those physicians. There's the sales call to the office. Companies also pay doctors to do industry research, for making positive speeches about their drugs at company-sponsored conferences, and for referring patients for clinical trials. Companies send them on free trips to exotic places, entertain them at dinners and at golf clubs, sport and theater events, bring free lunches to office staff, provide flashy handouts and thousands of samples, and may even offer to pay for their required continuing medical education (CME).

Doctors say they are not influenced by pressures to provide company-branded medications. However, recent research indicated that as little as one free meal from a drug company can influence which medicines doctors prescribe for Medicare patients. Even a small gift can result in patients being prescribed the branded higher cost medication rather than the cheaper generic. It was calculated that an estimated $73 billion yearly could be saved if equivalent generics were prescribed instead of brand-name drugs, with patients saving about a third of the cost.[39]

A number of former pharmaceutical company sales reps have gone public on *YouTube* to reveal a host of industry practices that they found unacceptable or unethical while employed in the industry. *YouTube* revelations began years ago and continue to this day.

Under a new federal healthcare transparency law called the Physician Payment Sunshine Act, drug and equipment makers must now disclose compensations, gifts and any so-called "transfers of value" they make to physicians or teaching hospitals. Some companies have reduced them, while others have not.[40] The payments are huge. One year, industry reported that it had paid doctors and institutions *$3.5 billion* in just the first five months of one year.[41]

ANOTHER HIGHLY-SUCCESSFUL marketing technique is hyping drugs for use "off-label," prescribing them for purposes other than those approved by the FDA. Although it is legal for physicians and other healthcare professionals to prescribe drugs for uses that the FDA has not specifically approved them for, *promoting and marketing them for off-label use is not legal*. In spite of this, the sales technique appears to be widespread and has helped boost drugs, including fluoroquinolones, to blockbuster status.

Abbott Laboratories once paid a fine of *$1.6 billion* for illegally promoting an anti-seizure pill off-label, the result of a lawsuit brought by a whistleblower. But huge settlements don't seem to stop illegal practices. Abbott, for one, put aside *more than a billion dollars* one year to settle legal cases.[42]

Misdeeds by J&J were spotlighted in one lawsuit by persons who claimed that the company hid serious side effects that came from taking Levaquin, deliberately mislabeled and misbranded the drug, and played down harmful side effects for its own financial gain resulting in significant harm or death to Levaquin consumers. J&J has been the target of thousands of lawsuits claiming that the company did not adequately warn patients about the drug's dangers. The company has settled more than 1,000 Levaquin injury cases.[43]

GlaxoSmithKline paid $3 billion one year in the largest healthcare fraud settlement in U.S. history. The company pled guilty to marketing a number of drugs illegally for off-label use, giving false statements and obstructing a federal investigation, paying kickbacks to doctors, failing to include certain safety data in reports to the FDA, and, despite warnings on the FDA-approved label, suggested that one drug had cardiovascular benefits when they were really risks. There was also Medicaid fraud due to misreporting prices covered by agreements. Four whistleblowers, including former executives, shared in the monetary agreement.[44]

In another case, $2.3 billion was paid by Pfizer to the Department of Justice. The company pled guilty to misbranding drugs with the intent to defraud or mislead and was found to have promoted four drugs illegally.[45]

Public Citizen notes that criminal and civil penalties paid by industry totaled more than *$36 billion* in one nine-year period. This public watchdog accused drug companies of adopting illegal behavior as part of their business model.[46] In the first-half of one year, *$6.6 billion* in fines was paid by the pharmaceutical industry to federal and state governments.[47] Ninety-two companies finalized 373 settlements and paid fines.[48] More than half of all monetary penalties every year are for illegal marketing, bribery, overcharging government programs such as Medicaid, promoting off-label, and paying kickbacks to doctors and other caregivers.[49]

Effective treatments have been discovered with off-label use. Sometimes a drug may be medically rational and appropriate. However, there are no standards that require scientific support for promoting medications for non-approved usage. Seventy-three percent of drugs promoted off-label have little or no back-up evidence.[50] Patients who receive a prescription off-label are 54% more likely to experience an adverse drug reaction than patients who are prescribed a drug for approved use.[51]

THE HIGH COST of drugs is another current issue. Prescription costs are higher in the U.S. than in the rest of the industrialized world because America's health care system allows pharmaceutical companies to set their own prices. There is no negotiation on the cost of medicines, unlike in almost every other country. Companies can set whatever price they want, and they do.[52]

Even prices of generic drugs are soaring. The purpose of generic manufacturing is to create and provide lower-priced meds as soon as the original drugs end their exclusivity production period. They are chemically identical to the brand name drugs, equally effective and prescribed for the same purposes. But consumers and insurers saw the average price per prescription for 50 of the most popular generics go from $13.14 in one four-year period to $62.10, an increase of 373%. Some generic companies don't say why their prices are going up. Others cite raw materials shortages, consolidation in the industry (less competition so they can charge higher prices) and medical advancements that make replicating brand-name drugs more expensive. The latter goes unexplained.[53]

Peter B. Bach, a drug-cost expert with Memorial Sloan-Kettering Cancer Center in New York recommends more analysis, as happens in other countries, of drug company costs of production.[54] It's a fact that nine out of the ten top pharmaceutical companies spend more on marketing than they do on research and development. Many blockbuster drugs now sold at high prices initially grew out of research paid by government not by the drug makers.[55]

Behind the scenes, pharmaceutical companies may be controlling prices and keeping them high by using certain sales tactics such as "exclusive dealing" or "bundling." In exclusive dealing, arrangements are made in which a large drug purchaser agrees to buy all its requirements from one manufacturer, which blocks competing products from selling to that buyer. Bundling involves providing discounts on several products in the pharmaceutical's portfolio as an incentive for large purchases, which can result in prices that competitors are not able to match.[56]

It isn't only pharmaceutical companies who are charging high rates for pills. In 2018, FDA Commissioner Scott Gottlieb accused pharmacy benefit managers in a complex medical distribution chain of contracting secretly with health insurance plans to favor older, more costly drugs over newer approved biosimilars, which are less costly.[57]

Drug spending per capita in the U.S. is more than double that of other countries and has also doubled per person in the last 10 years. These figures are largely driven by brand-name prices that have been increasing at rates far beyond the consumer price index.[58] It is also due to high-powered marketing departments at major pharmaceutical companies that push profits before remedy. Some of the largest companies in the industry had operating profit margins of 26% to 42.6%, compared to American Airlines at 13.2% and Exxon at 3.7%, companies that are considered to be well-run and successful.[59]

Consider these statistics:

• Nearly 70% of Americans are on at least one prescription drug. Mayo Clinic.

• For every $1 pharmaceutical companies spend on Research and Development for a new drug, they spend $19 on advertising that drug. *British Medical Journal.*

• In the United States, the cost of prescription drugs rises 12% every year. *Weedist.*

• 1 in 4 senior citizens skip doses of their prescribed medications in an attempt to reduce the amount of money they have to spend on drugs. *Business2Community.*[60]

Faced with numerous shortages of critical medications and frequent price gouging by the pharmaceutical industry, a group of 500 major U.S. hospitals, including the Mayo Clinic, recently established their own not-for-profit generic pharmaceutical company seeking to ensure a reliable supply of essential medicines and avoid industry price spikes. The consortium plans to begin by producing 14 critical generic medicines, but must first get FDA approval. The key question is whether the new company will pass along cost savings to their patients or simply rely on the new organization to enhance their own bottom line.[61]

IT SEEMS SCANDALOUS that industry can charge such high prices when they also outsource parts of the manufacturing process to low-wage countries to greatly reduce costs. If you are prescribed an antibiotic in Europe or North America, it is almost certain that the active pharmaceutical ingredients (APIs) came from China, then are made into pills or capsules and packaged in India. In the past three decades, most drug manufacturing operations have been outsourced to countries where wages are low and regulation is weak. China now provides 80 to 90 percent of APIs. India is the largest producer of finished medicines. Some manufacturing has also moved to Pakistan, Bangladesh and Southeast Asia. The supply chains are complex and virtually impossible to trace since arrangements are considered trade secrets and little information is published.

The city of Hyderabad in southeastern India is one of the largest centers of bulk drug production in the world. When researchers examined effluent from a wastewater treatment plant that processes waste from some ninety drug manufacturers in a Hyderabad suburb, they *found concentrations of ciprofloxacin one thousand times higher than the dosage recommended for patients with serious bacterial infections. It was estimated that the manufacturers must be discarding 45 kilograms of ciprofloxacin a day, enough to treat 44,000 people.*

This kind of contamination finds its way into ground water and drinking water, adding to the worldwide antibiotic resistance problem. Similar wastewater concentrations have been found in effluent emitted from Chinese, Korean, Taiwanese, and

Pakistani factories. One lake in India that was once popular for swimming and fishing has been described as "a giant Petri dish for anti-microbial resistance."

WHAT TO DO

- Read the information sheet that your pharmacist gives you with your prescription. But read with skepticism. Does it look like information might have been omitted? Are there important risks listed that require further research?

- Listen carefully to television advertising. Does it seem too good to be true? Does it compare itself favorably to other similar medications without showing proof? Do the ads say whether patients or doctors are actors or real people?

- Contact Public Citizen to learn more about pharmaceutical industry activities, good and bad, that affect your medications and their safety. www.publiccitizen.org.

- Be aware of drug marketing and promotions that seem overblown and may be untruthful.

- Get all the information you can about a drug before taking it and risking serious adverse reactions.

- Discuss drug costs with your pharmacist, insurer, hospital and nursing home to see if they can be lowered. You'd be surprised how many times this works.

- Consult the guide *Worst Pills, Best Pills*, authored by doctors, for comprehensive information about hundreds of drugs, their benefits and risks.

Big Pharma is regulated by the FDA, which is charged with the responsibility to approve new prescription drugs that are effective and safe for everyone. The agency is charged to protect us from taking harmful medications. But does it do that? Research indicates another side to the story.

Notes

1   "Too Many Meds." *Consumer Reports*, cover story, September 2017.

2   Petersen, Melody. *Our Daily Meds*, Picador, New York, NY, 2008, pp. 115-17.

3   Hughes, Jill Elaine. "Seeking magic in a bottle; Patent medicines promised cures but often delivered dangerous drugs." *Chicago Tribune*, May 5, 2013.

4   Hilts, Philip J. Protecting America's Health, The University of North Carolina Press, Chapel Hill and London, 2003, pp. 106-7.

5   Marchant, Jo. "When antibiotics turn toxic." *Nature*, March 21, 2018.

6   www.wikipedia.org.

7   "Quinolones Market to Undertake Strapping Growth by the End 2025." *Technology Market*, June 5, 2019.

8   Noah, Timothy. "The Make-Believe Billion; How drug companies exaggerate research costs to justify absurd profits." *Slate Magazine*. www.slate.com.

9   Almashat, Sammy, MD, MPH. "Pharmaceutical Research Costs: The Myth of the $2.6 Billion Pill." *Health Letter, Public Citizen*, September 2017.

10   Noah, Timothy. "The Make-Believe Billion; How drug companies exaggerate research costs to justify absurd profits." www.slate.com.

11   Scott, Anna. "Live Q&A: Funding drug development for diseases of poverty." *The Guardian*, March 27, 2014.

12   "Pharma Companies Buying Old Drugs, Dramatically Increasing Prices." *Worst Pills Best Pills Newsletter*, August 2015.

13   Almashat, Sammy, MD, MPH. "Pharmaceutical Research Costs: The Myth of the $2.6 Billion Pill." *Health Letter,* Public Citizen, September 2017.

14   Miller, Henry I. "Critics of 'Me Too Drugs' Need to Take a Chill Pill." *The Wall Street Journal,* January 1, 2014.

15   Angus, Ian. "Superbugs in the Anthropocene, A Profit-Driven Plague." *Monthly Review,* June 1, 2019.

16   Young, Robin and Hobson, Jeremy. "The Search for New Antibiotics." National Public Radio (NPR), February 17, 2014.

17   Light, Donald W. *The Risks of Prescription Drugs.* The Columbia University Press and Social Science Research Council Series on the Privatization of Risk, New York, NY, 2010, pp. 15-16.

18   Piller, Charles. "FDA and NIH clinical trial sponsors keep results secret and break the law." *Science,* January 13, 2020.

19   Seife, Charles, MS. "Research Misconduct Identified by the US Food and Drug Administration, Out of Sight, Out of Mind, Out of the Peer-Reviewed Literature." *JAMA,* February 9, 2015.

20   Gaensly, Joseph. "Oppositions Filed Against Gilead Hepatitis C Patent Applications in India." *Intellectual Property Watch,* July 20, 2018.

21   "Pharma Should Be Open About Money to Patient Groups." www.drugwatch.com.

22   www.opensecrets.org/news/2017.

23   "Pharmaceuticals/Health Products/Industry Profile: Summary, 2017." www.opensecrets.org.

24   "Pharmaceutical Manufacturing/Top Contributors, 2017-2018." www.opensecrets.org.

25   Aladdin, Meena, MS, PhD. "Companies Are Reaping Benefits from Social Influencers, and Big Pharma Wants In." *Health Letter,* March 2019.

26 "The 2017 DTC Report: All the data in one place." *Medical Marketing & Media*, March 29, 2017.

27 Tanner, Lindsey. "Medical marketing hits $30B." *Chicago Tribune, Associated Press*, January 10, 2019.

28 Angus, Ian. "Superbugs in the Anthropocene, A Profit-Driven Plague." *Monthly Review*, June 1, 2019.

29 Angus, Ian. "Superbugs in the Anthropocene, A Profit-Driven Plague." *Monthly Review*, June 1, 2019.

30 Carome, Michael, MD. "Outrage of the Month: Peddling Bad Medicine with Deceptive Advertising." *Health Letter, Public Citizen*, October 2014.

31 Carome, Michael MD. "Outrage of the Month: False and Misleading TV Drug Ads." *Health Letter*, Public Citizen, December, 2013.

32 McCafferty, Kevin. "PhRMA criticizes the FDA's research into drug advertising and promotion." *Medical Marketing & Media*, August 17, 2017.

33 Russell, John. "FDA: Ads carry risk of excessive warnings." *Chicago Tribune*, September 6, 2015.

34 Healy, David. Pharmageddon. *University of California Press*, Berkeley and Los Angeles, California, 2012, p. 260.

35 "VYVANSE for Binge Eating: Old Pill, New 'Disease'." *Worst Pills Best Pills Newsletter*, September 2015.

36 "Too Many Meds." *Consumer Reports*, cover story, September 2017.

37 "Big Pharma's Self-Promoting Media Campaign." *Worst Pills Best Pills Newsletter*, April 2017.

38 Rockoff, Jonathan D. "J&J Hires Chief Design Officer." *The Wall Street Journal*, March 19, 2014.

39 "Study: Even one free meal can sway doctors." *Portland Press Herald, Associated Press*, June 21, 2016.

40   Ornstein, Charles et al. "As sunshine law nears, Big Pharma trims." *Chicago Tribune*, March 5, 2014.

41   Loftus, Peter. "Doctors Net Billions From Drug Firms." *The Wall Street Journal*, October 1, 2014.

42   Frost, Peter. "Abbott settles Depakote case." *Chicago Tribune*, May 8, 2012.

43   Wasserman, Emily. "Levaquin users slap J&J with $800M RICO suit, claiming pharma giant hid serious side effects." www.fiercepharma.com, January 21, 2016.

44   Gotzsche, Peter C. *Deadly Medicines and Organised Crime.* Radcliffe Publishing, London, 2013, pp. 27-28.

45   Ibid, p.26.

46   "Drug Company CEOs: Rewarded For Illegal Acts?" *Worst Pills Best Pills Newsletter*, August 2013.

47   "Settlements for Prosecution of Fraud by Big Pharma at Record High." *Worst Pills Best Pills Newsletter*, November 2012.

48   Almashat, Sammy, MC, MPH. "Pharmaceutical Industry Continues to Defraud Federal, State Governments." *Health Letter*, Public Citizen, April 2016.

49   "Coverage of Supplements and Drugs: Fair and Balanced?" NCI Well Connect Mid-Week Brief, Nutritional Concepts, March 26, 2014.

50   Gulfo, Joseph V. "Ending the Prescribe-Don't-Tell Charade for Off-Label Drugs." *The Wall Street Journal*, March 27, 2016.

51   "New Evidence That Off-Label Drug Use Increases Risk of Harm." *Worst Pills Best Pills Newsletter*, January 2016.

52   Burton, Thomas M. "Trump Moves to Cut Costs for Prescription Drugs." *The Wall Street Journal*, February 9, 2018.

53   Hirst, Ellen Jean. "Why are the prices of generic drugs soaring?" *Chicago Tribune*, November 23, 2014.

54   Burton, Thomas M. "Trump Moves to Cut Costs for Prescription Drugs." *The Wall Street Journal*, February 9, 2018.

55   "Health-Care System Burdened by Soaring Drug Prices." *The Wall Street Journal*, Letters, July 27 2015.

56   Sinha, Michael S., MD, JD, MPH et al. "Antitrust, Market Exclusivity and Transparency in the Pharmaceutical Industry." *JAMA*, May 7, 2018.

57   Edney, Anna. "FDA head blasts drug supply chain as 'rigged.'" *Portland Press Herald*, Bloomberg Businessweek, March 8, 2018.

58   "Study examines reasons for high cost of prescriptions drugs in US, approaches to reduce costs." The JAMA Network Journal, August 23, 2016.

59   "Why Drugs Cost So Much." AARP Bulletin/Real Possibilities, May 2017.

60   Rapp, Adam. "10 Big Pharma Statistics That Will Make You Cringe." www.emedcert.com, July 13, 2016.

61   "Hospitals Band Together to Bypass Big Pharma, Start Their Own Drug Company." *Worst Pills Best Pills Newsletter*, November 2018.

COMPLEXITIES AT THE FDA

*The FDA acts essentially as an auditor
for drug company data and no more.*

DAVID HEALY, *PHARMAGEDDON*

WHO IS RESPONSIBLE for protecting us from the potential dangers of prescription drugs such as fluoroquinolones? In the United States it is the Food and Drug Administration (FDA), which operates under the Health and Human Resources Department. The mission of this regulatory agency is:

> to be responsible for protecting the public health by ensuring the safety, efficiency and security of human and veterinary drugs, biological products and medical devices and to ensure the safety of our nation's food supply, cosmetics and products that emit radiation.[1]

This is a huge agenda! Here is what the FDA states that it is doing to provide safety for our drugs, including fluoroquinolones:

It is the FDA's responsibility to determine whether a drug is safe and effective and the benefits of use outweigh the risks when used as intended and labeled.[2]

AN FDA COMMISSIONER is appointed by the President. Appointments may reflect more political intent than medical qualification. Tom Marciniak, a former FDA medical team leader, said: "You don't survive as a senior official at the FDA unless you are pro-industry. The FDA has to pay attention to what Congress tells them to do, and the industry will lobby to get somebody else in there if they don't like you."[3]

Unfortunately, this bureau has a checkered history of the kind of ethical issues that have been described as the FDA "getting into bed with industry." The FDA calls it a partnership. Henry Welch, director of the FDA's antibiotics division in the 1960s and an outspoken supporter of industry, was forced to resign when it was revealed that he had received more than $260,000 in payments from companies he was supposed to regulate.[4]

The regulator has consistently had to work with a limited budget and charges fees to speed up review of drug approval applications, which some consider a conflict of interest. An industry that is seeking approval for their drugs is funding an agency that grants those approvals. The FDA receives more than $1 billion annually from those fees.[5]

Public Citizen has criticized the FDA for nearly 50 years for approving new medications when available evidence demonstrated risks of serious harms that outweighed benefits. This advocate organization also has raised alarms about a federal agency that allows approved drugs to remain on the market when serious risks have been shown to exist.

IN SPITE OF ethical issues, here's how it works:

Once a drug is created by a pharmaceutical company, the developer has to submit data to the FDA about the medication's benefits, risks, ingredients, and outcomes of its clinical trials, as well as all information it has relating to the safety and efficacy of that drug. Industry wants approval, so it may, and frequently does, present data that shows the many *benefits* of its drug but de-emphasizes or includes little about the *risks* uncovered in clinical trials.

The FDA organizes an advisory committee to review all the data provided by the manufacturer. This can include thousands of pages of material. Members frequently only review a detailed summary that has been provided. Then it is up to advisors to decide whether to recommend the medication for approval and sale, or not.

Advisory committees are made up of doctors, scientists, educators and other experts. They have almost always received payments at one time or another from drug companies for research, writing articles about drugs, speaking at industry conferences, referring patients for trials and more. Even so, most deny that they will provide a biased review.

The FDA, instead of seeking independent experts, simply asks committee members to declare whether they have any conflicts of interest.[6] There are claims that it's impossible to get the expertise needed unless the FDA accepts conflicted committee members.[7] It seems that most experts have industry connections. One journalist contacted a society of rheumatologists to locate a doctor for an interview who wasn't being paid by any companies selling Vioxx or Celebrex, drugs that were causing heart attacks. *She was told that there were none that didn't have that industry connection.*[8] Despite this, there are leading academicians and other medical experts available who do not take money from industry who could serve as unbiased professionals, even though they are fewer in numbers.

In addition, the agency has been known to put pressure on advisors to alter negative conclusions in favor of a drug's approval, standard practice according to Dr. Peter Gotzsche. a leading expert in clinical trials and regulatory affairs.[9] Gotzsche says:

"I have great respect for the work conscientious scientists do at drug agencies. They have prevented many useless and harmful drugs from being approved and have withdrawn many from the market. However, they work in a system that is fundamentally flawed and where the benefit of doubt protects companies and not patients."[10]

Even after conclusions have been submitted, decisions can be reversed. Committee chairs in the past have actually ignored a panel's conclusion recommending no approval and allowed applications to be accepted anyway. In one instance, the chief of the FDA's antibiotics division received more than $250,000 in fees from companies whose antibiotics he was responsible for certifying and consequently reversed decisions on some of those drugs.[11]

The Edmond J. Safra Center for Ethics has presented evidence that about 90% of all new drugs approved by the FDA over a 30-year period were little or no more effective for patients than existing drugs. All, however, were more effective than placebos, pills with no effective health benefits at all.

PAPERWORK SUBMITTED FOR FDA drug approval is complicated. Pharmaceutical companies know how to intentionally present complex materials that may or may not be read and how to downplay risks that may have shown up in clinical trials. Trial data presented for new drugs has been found to be consistently *misreported*, *misconstrued*, *manipulated*, or *withheld*. Data is left out of applications if it is too negative. Pages have been found missing, and whole trials are sometimes omitted, says one reviewer.[12]

When medical journals published articles on 33 new drug applications, it was found they didn't present the same information that was submitted to the FDA.[13] Professional journals are perused by physicians and other caregivers who expect articles to be truthful and complete.

For an agency that is required to approve and monitor the safety of our drugs, it is disturbing to read that 70% of

FDA scientists surveyed said that they were not confident that products approved by the FDA were safe.[14]

"The way FDA approaches safety is to virtually disregard it," said former FDA Associate Director of the Office of Drug Safety David Graham in Congressional testimony. "FDA believes there is no risk that cannot be managed in the post-marketing setting," he said.[15] The post-marketing setting is where the FDA might require more studies, label changes or issuance of warnings, all after approval and as the product continues to be sold.

Those studies after approval are commonly ignored by industry. Only one-third of them are carried out. Some companies are so slow in conducting additional investigations that they complete them *after the drug has gone off patent years later*.[16] If done at all, they may be only observational reviews that won't detect signals of harm.[17]

Additional required trials are not closely monitored. Once again, in reality, the patient becomes the guinea pig. Those post-marketing studies are conducted by the companies themselves, by the way, not independent researchers, which leaves room for possible misconduct.

ONCE A DRUG is on the market, there may be notifications to the FDA of serious adverse effects that have occurred from taking that medication. Fluoroquinolones have consistently been reported to the FDA about harm and injury.

Adverse event data on Levaquin began in **1997**. Reports totaled 21,932 by the end of **2018**, including 668 deaths. Cipro reporting began in **1983** and rose to 11,401 submissions plus 302 deaths by **2018**. Avelox disclosures began in **1997** and totaled 14,159 complaints as well as 571 deaths in the same time period. Almost all accounts were considered serious or disabling. Those 47,492 reports concerning just three fluoroquinolones were sent to the FDA for 21 to 35 years following their approval. These figures reflect only a small portion of actual harmful events that probably occurred.[18]

If the bureau receives enough notifications of serious or life-threatening risks, it may issue an announcement called a black box warning. This is an alert noting newly-detected serious risks associated with that drug and is meant to warn physicians, hospitals, pharmacies, caregivers and others who prescribe or distribute drugs, as well as patients who take them. The FDA has to receive significant numbers of adverse events reports to issue a warning. These accounts come from patients, doctors and the pharmaceutical companies.

Hundreds of warnings are issued by the FDA every year and they may or may not be noted by medical professionals or even patients. Symptoms of an adverse event that could be due to the medication are in the paperwork provided to a patient when a prescription is filled at the pharmacy. Black box warnings are in there. Patients rarely read them.

Drug companies are required to report any adverse events that have been submitted to them. When Big Pharma receives such a notification from a physician or from any other source, it must report it to the

FDA within 15 days. However, reporting is sometimes delayed for weeks or months or not reported at all. Researchers analyzed more than 1.6 million cases of serious adverse effects that had been reported from 2004 to 2014. They discovered that 10%, including 40,000 that involved a patient death, were not sent to the FDA within the required 15-day window.[19]

Ria Redberg, editor-in-chief of *JAMA Internal Medicine*, observed: "Such reporting delays should never occur, as they mean more patients are exposed to potentially avoidable serious harm, including death." The FDA has the authority to withdraw approval of a prescription medicine if its manufacturer fails to report adverse events, but the delay tactic can save them from such action.[20]

According to the FDA:

An adverse drug reaction, also called a side effect, is any undesirable experience associated with the use of a medicine in a patient. Adverse events can range from mild to severe. Serious adverse events are those that can cause disability, are life-threatening, result in hospitalization or death or are birth defects.

The first year Levaquin was in circulation, J&J turned in 35 adverse event reports. Fourteen (40%) were accounts of death, required intervention, or were life-threatening. Hospitalization was necessary in 12 more cases (34%). The company's reports became less and less serious as the year went by with patient outcomes becoming noted simply as "other."

In **2008**, after numerous revelations of harm, injury and death, the FDA issued a black box warning for all fluoroquinolones citing increased risk of tendonitis and tendon rupture. Risk further increased in patients over 60, in patients taking corticosteroids and patients with kidney, heart or lung transplants. It called special attention to damage that could affect the Achilles tendon, rotator cuff, hand, biceps, or thumb.

Reports analyzed between January and March of **2011** produced another alert for all drugs in this class to warn of *pseudotumor cerebri*. This disorder produces pressure inside the head that can swell the optic nerve and result in vision loss.[21] An FDA drug surveillance review the following year, **2012**, disclosed that retinal detachment was yet another possible side effect of taking fluoroquinolones.[22]

A new black, box warning was issued in **2014** indicating serious adverse reactions including tendonitis, tendon rupture, peripheral neuropathy, central nervous system effects and exacerbation of myasthenia gravis, a weak muscle disease that can cause drooping eyelids and difficulty swallowing or chewing.[23]

Again in **2014**, the FDA issued an *expanded black box warning* adding information about risks to nerves and the central nervous system that included painful or burning sensations, tingling, numbness and other abnormal sensations, weakness, psychosis, paranoia, hallucinations, anxiety, confusion, depression, insomnia, dizziness, tremors, and severe headaches. The new alert further warned that all of these reactions might occur in the patient at the same time and reactions might be disabling and irreversible.[24]

Charles Bennett, MD, PhD, led an effort in **2015** to request that the FDA add possible mitochondrial (cell) toxicity and serious psychiatric events" to fluoroquinolone black box warnings. Bennett heads one of the largest and most successful pharmaceutical watchdog groups in the country, the Southern Network on Adverse Reactions (SONAR) that uses patient stories instead of data bases in its research. He is also an endowed chair in medication safety and efficacy at South Carolina College of Pharmacy. Bennett has linked fluoroquinolones to diseases such as Parkinson's, Alzheimer's, and amyotrophic lateral sclerosis (ALS or Lou Gehrig's Disease).[25]

In November **2015**, the FDA convened a panel of experts who described an ever-worsening series of health problems with Levaquin. Rachel Brummert, executive director of the Quinolone Vigilance Foundation, was one of more than 30 people who spoke during the open public hearing portion of the meeting about how these drugs had impacted their lives.

"I am living proof that the risks in using a fluoroquinolone to treat a routine infection far outweigh the benefits," she stated. She described the 10 ruptured tendons and progressive nerve damage she had suffered from taking Levaquin for a suspected sinus infection nine years earlier. She applauded the FDA for making patient safety a priority and added: "Curbing unnecessary prescribing of fluoroquinolones will save thousands of Americans from needless suffering."[26]

It was that same year, **2015**, that the FDA voted to recognize Fluoroquinolone Associated Disability (FQAD) as a syndrome, a condition characterized by a set of associated symptoms. The designation was based on 178 cases that the agency believed were clear-cut: *otherwise heathy people who took fluoroquinolones for minor ailments developed disabling and potentially irreversible conditions*. The FDA also noted at the same time that these drugs had a much higher percentage of disabilities than other antibiotics.[27]

Yet another black box warning was issued in **2017** advising that fluoroquinolones should *only be used as a last resort antibiotic*. Based upon new reports, the FDA also recommended that doctors not prescribe any of these pills to patients who have other treatment options for common ailments such as acute chronic bronchitis, COPD, acute uncomplicated bladder infection and acute sinusitis.[28]

Public Citizen requested that this last warning include an alert about the higher risk of life-threatening abnormal heart rhythms when taking Cipro, Levaquin and Avelox. The FDA, however, did not heed its advice.[29] Public Citizen also asserted that victims who reported adverse reactions after taking fluoroquinolones had symptoms lasting an average of 14 months. The longest duration of dire consequences was nine years.[30]

In July of **2018**, a safety warning from the FDA pointed to *dangerous drops in blood sugar and neurological side effects that could cause delirium and memory problems*. Low blood glucose levels induced by these antibiotics could result in health problems, including *coma*, especially among older people. Those with diabetes who are on medications to reduce blood glucose are also at risk, the FDA warned. [31]

At the end of **2018**, the FDA sent out yet another alert about fluoroquinolone risk that could cause *ruptures or tears of the aorta blood vessel.*[32] This very serious condition, called an aneurysm, can result in death. By now, these medications had been on the market for years and had multiple warnings issued about serious and even life-threatening consequences.

Even in the wake of all these warnings, a new fluoroquinolone was approved by the FDA in 2017. It's called Baxdela. The scientific name is *delafloxacin*. Clinical trials involved 1,042 patients in eastern Europe, South America and Asia with acute bacterial skin and skin structure infections (ABSSSI). Results demonstrated that this new drug *was not inferior* to other potent drugs such as vancomycin and aztreonam. The product was approved with the requirement that its label must include a boxed warning. The manufacturer was also ordered to conduct U.S. surveillance studies for five years to determine whether bacterial resistance develops.[33]

How does the FDA communicate black box warnings to doctors, nurses, pharmacists and other health care professionals? They send what are called "Dear Doctor Letters" that detail new and important drug information and indications. A review led by a University of Chicago professor on the effectiveness of these notifications found that FDA warnings and other communications had a mixed or unpredictable record of changing prescribing practices. Many of the FDA communications appeared to have had little or no effect at all.[34]

The FDA has no authority to require companies to recall a prescription drug because of potential contamination or other serious safety problems. The agency can only exert mandatory recall for infant formula, food, medical devices, biologic products (blood products, for example) and tobacco.[35] It can, however, request that a company voluntarily recall a defective drug from the marketplace.[36]

Rep. Rosa DeLauro (D-Conn) is trying to change that. She serves on the U.S. House committee that oversees the FDA. She wants the agency to mandate that prescription drugs be removed from the market when they are defective or dangerous.

"It's unconscionable that FDA is unable to recall potentially life-threatening medicines," she says.

The FDA puts off requesting voluntary withdrawal, sometimes for years, in order to "substantiate evidence and concern about public health," an agency representative said. The powerful pharmaceutical lobby also influences those decisions.

"About the agency DeLauro notes: "It's a consistent pattern. Anything that comes into question, their approach is [to] leave it on the market. In the meantime, let's do a little here, a little there, see where it goes."

The FDA can receive hundreds of reports of health problems with a drug, but after issuing safety warnings, it has no authority to order stores to remove the product or to require websites to stop offering it. Once the manufacturer receives an FDA request to voluntarily remove the pills from the market, it doesn't have to do it.[37]

ONE WEEK AFTER the September 11 terrorist attacks, there was an anthrax scare in Washington, DC. Letters containing deadly anthrax spores were mailed to several major news media offices and to two Senators, killing five people and infecting at least 68 others.[38] At many post offices, envelopes were handled or opened by employees who became dizzy or disoriented or experienced numbness and other serious medical manifestations.

Cipro was rushed into action. It had been stockpiled by the government in case of biological terrorism and was thought to be an antidote for anthrax poisoning. Weeks later adverse reactions began to appear in people taking Cipro. The quick issuance of this fluoroquinolone began to be questioned. Cipro was withdrawn but damage had already been done. Some of those affected recovered, some continued to have troubling symptoms and adverse effects.

According to Vincent Quagliarello, MD, clinical director of infectious diseases at Yale University School of Medicine, Cipro's effectiveness for anthrax poisoning is iffy. "Theoretically," he says, "Cipro should work in an anthrax attack, but it's never been tested, so no one really knows the optimal dose or therapy or even, for sure, that it works at all." Taking Cipro for anthrax poisoning would have been considered an off-label treatment. Still, the risk was taken.[39]

IN NOVEMBER 2016, the FDA held a hearing to gather input for changing the agency's rules limiting off-label promotion, which had been requested by industry. Companies claimed that the First Amendment allowed them to distribute sales materials and publish in medical journals about off-label treatment for uses that had not been approved by the FDA.

Experts from Public Citizen and more than two dozen drug safety advocates presented data to show that for 80% of cases when a drug is prescribed for an unapproved use, there is a lack of evidence that it is effective and a patient is more likely to experience an adverse reaction. Thousands of patients, they reported, had serious and debilitating injuries from fluoroquinolones that were prescribed for off-label use. Public Citizen pointed to the FDA's public health imperative to provide effective and safe products. The group further warned that the FDA's decision on this matter could have profoundly dangerous consequences and undermine the entire FDA process.[40] No action was taken.

On a positive note, the FDA severely criticized several large drug makers for withholding samples of drugs from generic manufacturers after patents had expired. Generic companies require from 1,000 to 5,000 pills to identify a brand's active ingredients in order to reproduce generic versions. The delay tactic by holders of patents costs patients, insurers, and government programs more than $6 billion.[41]

In 2018, FDA Commissioner Scott Gottlieb announced that he would publish a list of companies that have potentially tried to forestall competition from generic alternatives, saying that companies need to "end the shenanigans." He also stated that the FDA would continue to work on this issue with the Federal

Trade Commission (FTC), whose mission is to police anti-competitive behavior.[42]

In a disturbing reversal, the FDA has announced withdrawal of a proposed ruling that would have asked generic drug companies to immediately update safety warnings on their product labels, a procedure that brand-name drug companies had been able to do for decades. Generic companies objected that updating safety warnings would cause significant new burdens and costs. Consequences of that action are that many of the new warnings about fluoroquinolones and other drugs may not be updated on generic products or in their guidance materials.[43]

WHAT TO DO

- Do not use any newly FDA-approved drug until it has been on the market for several years and is less likely to be the subject of a safety withdrawal or a black box warning.

- If Big Pharma advertising claims FDA approval, you can confirm this claim by searching for FDA-approved drugs at www.fda.gov

- If you have had an adverse event after taking a fluoroquinolone or any other drug, report it promptly to the FDA's online Med Watch site. Access this website at www.accessdata. fda.gov/scripts/medwatch. Or phone

1-800-FDA-1088 to report an event or injury or request that a form be mailed to you.

- Stay alert to new warnings on drugs that your physician is prescribing or that you are currently taking. Access www.fda.gov/drugs/postmarket-drug-safety-information-patients-and-providers/index-drug-specific-information and search for the name of your drug. Or, simply ask your physician to look it up in his or her online Physician's Desk Reference (PDR).

- If you think you may have had an adverse reaction to a fluoroquinolone or any other drug, discuss it with your doctor as soon as possible. If it seems highly likely, or confirmed, that a medicine has made you ill, request that your physician report your case to the FDA. The reporting system is designed to call attention to drug safety for patients as well as alert the medical community.

ONCE THE FDA has approved a drug, it will be marketed, sold and distributed. It will be available not only for prescription by doctors, but also distributed to patients in hospitals and by pharmacies, nursing homes and other businesses and organizations that provide care and systems for the ill, injured or elderly. These establishments are responsible for managing the dispensing of those medications wisely and safely. Research indicates that this is not always the case.

Notes

1   www.fda.gov/about-fda/what-we-do.

2   IBID.

3   Carome, Michael, MD. "Outrage of the Month: Agency Insiders Recount FDA's Cozy Relationship with Industry." *Health Letter,* August 2018.

4   Angus, Ian. "Superbugs in the Anthropocene, A Profit-Driven Plague." *Monthly Review,* June 1, 2019.

5   Carome, Michael, MD. "Outrage of the Month: Agency Insiders Recount FDA's Cozy Relationship with Industry." *Health Letter,* August 2018.

6   Gotzsche, Peter C. *Deadly Medicines and Organised Crime.* Radcliffe Publishing Ltd, London, p. 109.

7   Ibid, p.108.

8   Ibid, p.169.

9   Ibid. p.33.

10   Ibid, p.107.

11   Ibid, p.113.

12   Ibid, p.120.

13   Ibid, p.137.

14   Ibid, p.110.

15   Ibid, p.110.

16   Ibid, p.173.

17   Ibid, p.110.

18   www.fda.gov.

19 "Drug Industry's Unacceptable Delays in Reporting Adverse Events to the FDA." *Worst Pills, Best Pills Newsletter*, November 2015.

20 Ibid.

21 www.fda.gov/Drugs/ GuidanceComplianceRegulatoryInformation.

22 "Fluoroquinolone Antibiotics Associated with Increased Risk of Retinal Detachment." *Worst Pills Best Pills Newsletter*, July 2012.

23 www.fda.gov/news-events/pressannouncements/ fda-update-warnings-fluoroquinolone-antibiotics.

24 www.fda.gov/drugs/drug-safety-and-availability.

25 Danielson, Ryne. "RX warning: Possible side effects from some antibiotics." *Newsroom*, Medical, University of South Carolina, April 7, 2015.

26 Carr, Teresa. "Fluoroquinolones Are Too Risky for Common Infections."*Consumer Reports*, May 16, 2016.

27 Marchant, Jo. "When antibiotics turn toxic." *Nature*, March 21, 2018.

28 www.fda.gov.

29 Ibid.

30 "FDA Requires Stronger Warnings for Commonly Used Antibiotics." *Worst Pills, Best Pills Newsletter*, February 2017.

31 "FDA Requires Safety Label Changes for Fluoroquinolones." *HealthDay News*, July 11, 2018.

32 www.fda.gov/drugs/drug-safety-and-avilability.

33 Volker, Rebecca, MSJ. "Another Fluoroquinolone Approved." www.jamanetwork.com, August 1, 2017.

34 Tobacman, Jessica. "FDA alerts record mixed U. of C. study finds." *Chicago Tribune*, February 15, 2012.

35 "A Dangerous Gap in FDA Recall Authority." *Worst Pills Best Pills Newsletter*, September 2014.

36 www.fda.gov/safety/recalls-market-withdrawals-safety-alerts.

37 Newkirk, Margaret and Berfield, Susan. "How Do You Stop Taking Recalled Medication If You Don't Know It's Been Recalled?" Bloomberg Businessweek, December 13, 2019.

38 "2001 Anthrax attacks." www.Wikipedia.org.

39 Lewin, Tamar. "A Nation Challenged: Fear of Infections; Anthrax Scare Prompts Run on an Antibiotic." The New York Times, September 27, 2001.

40 "Patient Safety Advocates, Industry Spar Over Off-Label Promotion." *Worst Pills Best Pills Newsletter*, January 2017.

41 Johnson, Linda A. "FDA names drugmakers accused of blocking cheaper generic drugs." *Portland Press Herald*, Associated Press, May 18, 2018.

42 "More Competition for Pharma." *The Wall Street Journal*, May 19, 2018.

43 www.fda.gov

HOSPITALS AND PHARMACIES:
CAREFUL OR CARELESS

Automatic prescribing of antibiotics in hospitals is common and often incorrect.

BETSEY MCCAUGHEY, *THE WALL STREET JOURNAL*

Speed in filling prescriptions, pressures to meet quotas, distractions, limited time to do safety checks and burnout contribute to the need for more pharmacy rules.

SAM ROE AND RAY LONG, *CHICAGO TRIBUNE*

WHEN YOU ARE admitted to a hospital, it is likely that you will be prescribed an antibiotic to prevent infection while under hospital care, although antibiotics are not formulated to prevent but to cure bacterial infection. Fluoroquinolones are one of the most commonly prescribed medications given in medical institutions. More and more hospitals, however, are instituting stewardship programs to reduce their use in consideration of antibiotic resistance, i.e. overuse that results in eventual ineffectiveness of those drugs.

Fluoroquinolone overuse in the hospital setting appears to have been prevalent. These antibiotics have been given to patients whether there is bacterial infection or not. When given in one group of hospitals, 39% were administered for non-infectious or non-bacterial syndromes or given for longer than recommended. It resulted in more than a quarter of those patients suffering adverse effects.[1]

This kind of antibiotic overuse can lead to infectious bacteria resisting any cure at all and may lead to the acquiring of serious life-threatening diseases. These diseases occur primarily in hospitals or nursing homes. Germs that resist cure by even the most powerful drugs available are commonly called Superbugs. They kill an estimated 35,000 people in the US each year.[2]

INSTITUTIONALLY-ACQUIRED DISEASES go by the names *Clostridium Difficile (C. diff)*, *Methicillin-resistant Staphylococcus Aureus (MRSA)*, and colistin-resistant *Klebsiella Pneumoniae Carbapenemase (KPC)*. They are very difficult to treat when powerful antibiotics, such as Levaquin, may no longer work. Drug-resistant infections, are now the third leading cause of death in the United States, killing an estimated 162,000 people a year. The toll is far higher in Africa, Asia and Latin America.[3]

Symptoms of *C. diff* are watery diarrhea, severe abdominal pain, possible fever, nausea, loss of appetite and weight loss. It's serious business. The CDC has estimated that there have been 453,000 cases of *C. diff* that resulted in 29,300 deaths within 30 days of diagnosis. Josh Farkas writes on *PulmCrit*, a pulmonary and critical care website, that fluoroquinolones are well-known to cause *C. diff* infection.

After a large outbreak of this illness at the University of Chicago Hospital, it was found that extensive use of Levaquin had contributed substantially to the increase of patients with the infection. Farkas says that fluoroquinolones do not appear to be suitable for sustained use in hospitals as "workhorse" antibiotic therapy, that is, commonly used in numerous situations.[4]

MRSA, on the other hand, may attack your bones, joints, bloodstream, heart valves, lungs or recent surgical sites. The *S. aureus* in MRSA is a common bacterium that doesn't normally cause illness until it acquires resistance to antibiotics. Resistance in MRSA cases has been linked to the fluoroquinolones Cipro and ciprofloxacin.

Looking at MRSA hospital cases that occurred over more than 10 years, it was discovered that there was a significant drop in MRSA infection following reduction in the use of Cipro. When this antibiotic was eliminated, MRSA infections fell by half, from an average of about 120 a month to around 60. Improved cleaning and hand washing didn't figure in the decrease of infection rates. The only major change coincided with fewer Cipro prescriptions.[5]

MRSA is no longer confined to hospital settings. It has been reported that many cases are showing up outside of hospitals, sickening thousands of Americans with minor skin boils to deadly pneumonia and claiming upwards of 20,000 lives in communities of school children, soldiers, prison inmates, and even NFL players.[6]

SINCE UP TO 80% of every dose of an antibiotic is excreted unchanged, hospital waste products typically contain high concentrations of antibiotics and bacteria. If appropriate sewage treatment is available, some antibiotics may be eliminated but even advanced treatment systems do not remove resistant bacteria.[7]

Deadly antibiotic-resistant bacterium is increasingly found even in soil. Antibiotics are routinely given to farm animals for disease, infection prevention, or to create faster or fatter growth. Approximately 90% of these drugs end up being excreted as urine or manure, says Holly Dolliver, PhD, a professor of crop and soil sciences. Scientists at the University of Minnesota found antibiotic residues in corn, green onions, and cabbage after growing on soil fertilized with livestock manure.

Forty-five percent of Midwest hog farms studied had MRSA germs, according to University of Iowa researchers. They also reported that 64% of farm workers were MRSA carriers.[8] These deadly germs have also been found on Florida swimming beaches. They have been transported by farm trucks, farm workers, and houseflies. The inside air of a car that was simply following a poultry truck in traffic was tested and found to be filled with MRSA bacteria. Even the surface of an unopened soft drink can in that car was infected.[9]

A lethal community-based KPC once raced through the Health Medical Center in Bethesda, Md, and staff were unable to control its spread. A woman with lung disease had entered the hospital as a patient. When her chart indicated that she was a KPC carrier, the staff immediately isolated the patient and took all precautions to avoid contact and spread of disease. Weeks later patients began to come down with KPC. The only explanation was traced to the initial patient. Before the outbreak was finally contained, two patients had died. If you are a healthy individual, you have a low risk for contacting KPC or other such infections, but as people come to hospitals with other medical conditions, susceptibility is higher.[10]

Betsey McCaughey, former lieutenant governor of New York and founder and chair of the Committee to Reduce Infection Deaths, has suggested that the CDC make KPC a reportable disease, like AIDS. It would reveal how many cases there are and where they are in order to track this more recent dangerous infection.[11]

The U.S. Center for Infectious Diseases (CID) issued a warning about a growing world-wide threat from these infections. Canadian Medical Association (CMA) announced back in 2009 that it was concerned about the emergence of antibiotic resistant organisms and called it a major public health problem in hospitals and other health care settings.

Acquired-disease management and treatment options are limited. Drug resistant pathogens are appearing more frequently as new antibiotic discovery and development slows dramatically. CMA warns that "in the not-too-distant future, we may be faced with a growing number of potentially untreatable infections."[12]

Antibiotics that were once considered a miracle of modern medicine could contribute to a future global health crisis. Canada's Chief of Public Health has estimated that antibiotic resistant infections could cause 10 million deaths per year globally by 2050, more than the current annual worldwide deaths from cancer.[13] Miracle drugs are losing their magic.

ALMOST FROM THE time Levaquin was approved, it became the preferred antibiotic among more than half of all general medical-surgical hospitals in the US.[14] Fluoroquinolones prescribed in emergency department and ambulatory clinic visits during one seven-year period rose threefold, from use in 7 million visits to more than 22 million.[15]

When 111 patients in 36 hospitals were treated with antibiotics for UTIs, nearly 40% of them did not have testing or evaluation before those drugs were given.[16] It is well known in the medical community that these drugs should not be given when bacteria are not present, but testing takes time and doctors want to to provide immediate relief.

Nearly 60% of patients hospitalized for asthma are prescribed antibiotics, even though guidelines advise against prescribing in the absence of infection. About 40% admitted to hospitals were found to have been prescribed antibiotics on the first day even before evaluation had taken place.[17] Nearly half of all patients who go to urgent care clinics seeking treatment for conditions that don't require antibiotics received a prescription for one anyway, Lena H. Sun wrote in *The Washington Post*.[18]

ON A POSITIVE note, antibiotic stewardship is beginning to take hold in many hospitals. It includes training, revision of rules and procedures, pre-prescription approval, and feedback from peers in order to generate a reduction in the use of antibiotics when other effective medications could be given instead.

When fluoroquinolone prescribing for hospitalized patients who had pneumonia and UTIs was studied, results showed that institutions that had stewardship programs gave patients fewer of these powerful medications. The surprise statistic, however, was that 66% of fluoroquinolones prescribed occurred at discharge. It didn't make any difference whether hospitals were practicing stewardship or not.

Even more surprising, hospitals with stewardship programs that specifically targeted fl uo roquinolone use had an even higher prescription rate for them at discharge, more than 78%! Hospitalists were frequently prescribing these first-line antibiotics when the patient was ready to leave the hospital. Hospitalists are doctors who take the place of your personal doctor when you are admitted, make diagnoses, order labs and figure out which drugs to prescribe and send home with you. Neither doctors nor hospitals monitor drug use after a patient leaves the building, so there is no way to know if a patient actually takes his or her medication or completes the number of days recommended to take them.

"On a national level, we really should start to think about monitoring antibiotic prescribing that happens at discharge, not just during hospitalization," says researcher Valerie Vaughn, MD.[19]

Changes in prescribing habits are difficult to overcome despite the fact that awareness of serious adverse effects and antibiotic resistance is emerging. Prescribing of fluoroquinolones for off-label use is common even after warnings have been issued. Doctors are still prescribing their drugs at the same rate as in the past even as warnings and articles have been published about them being given unnecessarily.[20]

In the hospital Emergency Room (ER) inappropriate use of antibiotics has not decreased, according to results of a one-year research project. This is despite mounting concerns about their use and when stewardship programs have been initiated. ER personnel did limit use of antibiotics for acute respiratory infections in children, but there was no decrease in use for adults with the same infections. Fluoroquinolones are still being prescribed for sinusitis and bronchitis even when those infections are caused by a virus.[21]

Nursing home residents are the recipients of frequently prescribed antibiotics. Up to 70% receive one or more courses of them every year for UTIs, pneumonia, cellulitis or other conditions. Up to 75% of those prescriptions are given incorrectly. It may be the wrong drug, the wrong dose or the wrong duration. Or, they may be dispensed unnecessarily. One quarter to one third of people in nursing homes who are diagnosed with UTIs have no actual symptoms. Those suffering from dementia may be unable to tell nurses or doctors exactly what their symptoms are. The most common antibiotics given for UTIs are fluoroquinolones.

"UTIs are the poster child of inappropriate antibiotic use," says David Nace of the University of Pittsburgh.[22]

It's troubling to realize that antibiotic stewardship has been ongoing for more than 50 years with little improvement until recently. Hospitals are beginning to take another look at how to improve their facilities and practices to prevent infections. Institutions are changing the design of patient rooms, which have been altered little since World War II, to create an environment that minimizes the transmission of bacteria and adds more air circulation. Some have also added probiotics, such as yogurt, to the patient diet to better balance bacteria in the intestine. Hospitals that prescribed probiotics for a few days or up to three weeks reduced antibiotic-associated diarrhea by 60%.[23]

Some hospitals have tried to discourage the proliferation of resistant strains of bacteria by instituting a restricted list of commonly misused antibiotics such as fluoroquinolones. A doctor who prescribes one of the drugs on the list has to justify his selection to a member of the hospital's infectious diseases unit before the pharmacy will dispense. Disciplinary action is a last resort.[24]

HOSPITALS AS WELL as doctors rely increasingly on electronic health recordkeeping (EHR), which has seen its share of corporate fraud. Software vendors rushed to get the billions in subsidies that the federal government issued to encourage streamlining of medical records systems. In doing so, dozens of them cut corners and gamed the system so that they would qualify. Their systems were purchased by thousands of hospitals and physicians that trusted the software to keep accurate patient records. There have been glitches, however, that prevent doctors from accessing files quickly, that mix up patients and their medications, or send vital test results to the wrong file. Any of these can contribute to serious patient injury or even death. A number of companies have settled lawsuits. The technology has not been removed from the market. Hospitals and physicians find that it's difficult to switch to another product or remove such programs.[25]

Medical institutions have massive data in patients' digital health records. Some hospitals are beginning to share that data with large companies such as Microsoft, International Business Machines (IBM) and Amazon.com Inc. Digitizing patients' medical histories, lab results and diagnoses has created a booming market in which tech giants are looking to store and crunch medical data with potential for groundbreaking discoveries and lucrative products. Hospitals make efforts not to share personal data that would identify patients, but doctor notes may include such information and can be transmitted along with other data.

Hospitals can share patient data as long as they follow federal privacy laws, which contain limited consumer protections. Health information technologist Lisa Bari says: "The data belongs to whoever has it."[26]

THE PHARMACIST IS thought to be the last defense against being harmed by drugs. He or she would presumably notice if a prescription was potentially dangerous when they observe a customer's record of medications. A pharmacist would note if a prescription appears to be an inaccurate dosage or if it would interact dangerously with another medicine being taken. Doctors say they rely on pharmacists to check on those concerns. However, pharmacists also have work issues.

A pharmacist is authorized to ask a customer or a prescribing physician why a drug was ordered or why a certain dosage is prescribed if they are suspicious that there may be an error or the prescription doesn't seem to fit the diagnosis. But this takes time and there may be long lines waiting.

A growing trend is for pharmacy professionals to ignore flagged notifications in their computer systems that provide alerts. There are hundreds, even thousands, of warnings that have been issued over the years for a multitude of medicines. For pharmacists, the showing of warning after warning can easily cause "alert fatigue," as it has been called, or information overload. It causes pharmacists to simply turn off their flagging system, according to reports, resulting in missed warnings.[27]

An investigation by reporters at the *Chicago Tribune* covered visits to urban pharmacies as well as dispensaries located in smaller Illinois communities. They found that most pharmacists failed to discuss serious drug interactions when they presented them with prescriptions that were unsafe when taken together.[28]

A follow-up newspaper series about their visits resulted in a bill being introduced in the Illinois legislature that would restrict hours pharmacists can work each day, limit the number of prescriptions they can fill each hour, require break time, and provide whistleblower protection. Speed in filling prescriptions, overwhelming pressures to meet quotas, distractions, limited time to do safety checks, and burnout contribute to the need for new pharmacy rules, the reporters wrote.[29]

Pharmacists get prescriptions with misspellings, hurried handwriting or inaccurate input on computers. Dosages may be suspect, either too much or too little. Computer screening programs may detect these errors, although not every time apparently.

A report on *CBC Vancouver News* featured the case of a woman who died. A physician, two pharmacists and a computer system failed to detect warnings of a medicine interaction that foretold an adverse event. In this case, it was a shutdown of her immune system and ultimate death.

"One death is really the tip of the iceberg," says a University of Victoria drug policy researcher. "I think there are many hundreds, probably thousands of adverse drug reactions that happen [like this]."[30]

Georgetown University Medical Center ran a test at 50 pharmacies in the Washington, DC area. Test takers posed as customers and provided prescriptions for both Seldane and erythromycin, also dangerous drugs when taken together. One third of the pharmacy professionals filled the prescriptions without a word of caution or a call to the doctor. The person presenting the prescription asked pharmacists specifically if these two drugs should be taken together. The majority said there was no problem.

Reporters from *U.S. News and World Report* sent out reporters to confirm those findings. They presented three paired prescriptions at pharmacies for medications that shouldn't be taken together. Many filled the orders without comment. All but two pharmacies were using computer screening programs that detect errors in prescriptions or provide alerts about patient risk. Pharmacists are usually able to recognize mistakes without computer warnings if they are alert. But screening programs confirm those errors.

More than 60% of visits to a doctor end with a prescription being given, writes Stephen Fried in his book *Bitter Pills*. He recognized that more and more orders are being called in to the pharmacist or prescribed by computer without a doctor visit. Physicians are influenced by advertising and sales calls from pharmaceutical reps and will actually order by brand name rather than a scientific name, in effect prescribing a widely-promoted medication over a generic that might be available and less expensive.

Federal legislation introduced by Maine's Senator Susan Collins passed in 2018 that requires pharmacists to counsel customers on whether their purchase would be cheaper if they didn't use their insurance coverage. Prior to this, what is known as the "gag law" prevented pharmacies from giving out this information, causing patients to pay more out-of-pocket costs for drugs than they should. The law also prohibits insurers and pharmacy benefits managers from restricting information about cheaper options. Pharmacy benefits managers are middlemen that insurers pay to set up a list called a "formulary" designating which drugs will be covered by health insurance plans.[31]

Selected Canadian community pharmacies participated in a trial to determine if an "educational intervention" would make a difference in discontinuing inappropriate prescriptions for older adults. Pharmacists were encouraged to send elderly customers an educational brochure that suggested de-prescribing of inappropriate medications. They also sent their physicians an evidence-based opinion that recommended de-prescribing those same medicines. The patients' mean age was 75. Within six months, the intervention saw a reduction of inappropriate prescribing by 43% of the doctors.[32]

Community pharmacies, surprisingly, sometimes even provide pills without a prescription. According to a recent research project involving pharmacies worldwide, 78% were found to have provided prescriptions without a doctor's order when customers requested it. And 58% of the pharmacies sold drugs only upon their own recommendation. Fluoroquinolones were the most common antibiotics provided without a prescription order.[33]

THERE'S ANOTHER PROBLEM with the prescription flyers you receive at the pharmacy. You get one set of guidelines, and the doctor receives a different one. Both are incomplete and misleading, according to detailed reviews by researchers at the

Dartmouth Institute for Health Policy and Clinical Practice.

Results of those flyer inspections showed that information omitted data on benefits as well as risks that could impair decision-making. This was found not only in guidelines but on the drug's label as well. Benefits were overestimated while side effects were downplayed and included no details on trial frequency. Severe side effects were hidden among milder conditions or not included at all. Trial data that would be helpful to consumers or physicians for decision-making was omitted.

The researchers found this also to be true in Direct-To-Consumer advertising as well as in medical journals read by doctors. Benefits were magnified and harmful effects minimized or omitted. Proposed was a revised label and guidelines format for consumers that would include clear answers to questions. It would also add a new section.

- What is this drug for?

- Who might consider taking it?

- How long has the drug been used?

- What precautions should I take?

- What other choices are there?

- What difference did this drug make?

- What are the serious side effects
  and symptom side effects?

- Inclusion of a highlighted section on
  warnings about uncommon life-threatening
  and very serious side effects.

Revisions were suggested for both the consumer guidelines and labels as well as the physician version. Recommendations and a new label format were presented to the FDA, but the agency announced that it would need at least three to five years to make a decision. Given its potential public health impact, said the researchers, physicians and the public should not have to wait that long for better drug information.[34]

IN ADDITION TO these worries, there is a growing black market for stolen, counterfeit, or fake drugs that may end up in pharmacies, nursing homes, hospitals and doctors' offices. In one year, federal agents seized close to $73 million in counterfeit drugs, a tiny slice of illicit activities. The international drug black market was estimated at more than $200 billion in 2016 and accounted for 10% of the entire pharmaceuticals supply chain.

You run the risk of purchasing black market drugs when you order medications through internet pharmacies. The Government Accountability Office estimates that there are at least 36,000 rogue online drug ordering sites. Besides the possibility of buying meds that include too much, too little or no active ingredients, you may be getting meds that include dangerous contaminants. Some of those found in confiscated drugs include heavy metals, rat poison and even toxic highway paint. Eighty-five percent of sellers advertising themselves as Canadian pharmacies to project an air of legitimacy were found to be based in some 27 other countries.[35]

Buying on third party internet sites can be risky. You could be getting non-authentic products from unknown sellers. Medications may have been improperly stored or may be expired. Buyer beware. Purchase only from a certified pharmaceutical site.

BETSY LEHMAN, HEALTH columnist for *The Boston Globe*, would have written a great column about her case, had she lived to write about it. She was accidentally given a quadruple dose of a chemo drug to treat breast cancer at the renowned Dana Farber Cancer Institute. Chemo drugs can include powerful fluoroquinolones, although it is not known if they were given in this case. Two months after she died, the mistake was discovered. Her case eventually inspired new hospital pharmacy rules, additional supervision, and, more radically, a plan to listen more carefully to patient complaints about side effects. Lehman's symptoms, which appeared immediately after she was given the toxic dose, were shrugged off as a normal reaction.[36]

Drug-induced injuries are the fourth leading cause of death in hospital settings, reports David Healy in his book *Pharmageddon*. He speculates that drug injuries are possibly the greatest single source of disability in the developed world.

WHAT TO DO

- If possible, always have a relative, friend or other advocate with you at the hospital to observe what is happening, ask questions, and monitor your care.

- When drugs new to you are being administered, ask what they are and what they are for. Are they prescribed by your doctor or automatically given by the hospital? You can refuse to take them until you have answers you are comfortable with.

- Get to know what your meds look and taste like. If a nurse brings you something different than you have been taking, ask why. The nurse should look at your hospital wristband before giving you anything.

- At discharge, repeat instructions so that it is clear to you what you are to do or not do. Ask if you should continue to take medications you were taking before your hospitalization.[37]

- If at all possible, don't schedule surgery or hospitalization during the month of July. Studies have shown that 10 percent more hospital errors are made in that month. Speculation is that thousands of new doctors begin their residencies at teaching hospitals that month and they are less experienced.[38]

- Ask to see a complete printout of your hospital bill with all costs listed. If you find your bill has errors, you have been double-billed for items, or invoices seem overinflated or exceptionally high, ask the billing department to take another look at your charges and provide explanations or corrections.

- You can negotiate prices at many hospitals. Always ask. You can find a list of average prices for procedures and medications at www.healthcarebluebook.com.

- You might want to contact a financial advocacy company that can review your bill for errors or overcharges, such as Virginia-based Medical Billing Advocates of America, Boston-based CoPatient, or www.disputebills.com.

- If your loved one becomes a resident of a nursing home, ask to review the daily procedures and medications. If you have any questions whatsoever about safety, meds or schedules, speak up and get answers you are comfortable with. Review drug dosages and when they will be given. Contact his or her physician if you still have questions.

- Get to know your pharmacist and feel free to ask him or her any questions you may have about your prescriptions. You are allowed to ask your pharmacist or doctor to provide information provided only to health care professionals.

- Avoid small, independent pharmacies in large cities that sell drugs at cut-rate prices. They are likely to be offering either counterfeit, out-of-date, or unsafe products.

- Purchasing drugs on the internet is not wise when you can't confirm how they were obtained, if they are legitimate, or if they have passed inspections for purity. If you're shopping online, look for Verified Internet Pharmacy Practice sites that are listed at www.nabp.net.

INSTITUTIONAL SETTINGS AREN'T the only areas where there are questionable practices. Unhealthy situations have also invaded the patient's first line of care, the physician's office.

Notes

1   Werner, Nicole L., et al. "Unnecessary use of fluroquinolone antibiotics in hospitalized patients." www.biomedcentral.com, July 5, 2011.

2   Evans, Melanie. "Patients Often Get Antibiotics Without a Doctor Visit, Study Finds." *The Wall Street Journal*, February 3, 2020.

3   Angus, Ian. "Superbugs in the Anthropocene, A Profit-Driven Plague." *Monthly Review*, June 1, 2019.

4   Farkas, Josh. "Six reasons to avoid fluoroquinolones in the critically ill." *PulmCrit*, August 1, 2016.

5   Knight, Gwenan M., et al. "Shift in dominant hospital-associated methicillin-resistant Staphylococcus aureus clones over time." *Journal of Antimicrobial Chemotherapy*, October 2012, pp. 2514-2522.

6   Eisler, Peter. "Deadly, drug-resistant bug spreading beyond hospitals." *USA TODAY*, December 17, 2013.

7   Angus, Ian. "Superbugs in the Anthropocene, A Profit-Driven Plague." *Monthly Review*, June 1, 2019.

8   Rosenberg, Martha. *Born with a Junk Food Deficiency: How Flaks, Quacks, and Hacks Pimp the Public Health.* Prometheus Books, Amherst NY, 2012, p. 205.

9   Ibid, p.207.

10 A Large Outbreak of Clostridium Difficile-Associated Disease With An Unexpected Proportion of Deaths and Colectomies at a Teaching Hospital Following Increased Fluoroquinolones Use." *Infection Control and Hospital Epidemiology*, March 2005.

11 McCaughey, Betsey. "When Hospitals Become Killers." *The Wall Street Journal*, January 31, 2013.

12 Mulvey, Michael R., PhD and Simor, Andrew E., MD. "Antimicrobial resistance in hospitals: How concerned should we be?" *CMAJ*, February 17, 2009.

13   "Antimicrobial resistance 'future global health crisis' reports Canada's Public Health Officer. CMA releases new policy on AMR." *Canadian Medical Association*, www.cma.ca, June 16, 2019.

14   "Levaquin is the Preferred Quinolone Among More Than Half of All General Medical-Surgical Hospitals in the United States." *PR Newswire*, December 2, 2008.

15   Linder, J.A. et al. "Fluoroquinolone prescribing in the United States: 1995-2002." Brigham and Women's Hospital, and Harvard Medical School, Boston, Mass., abstract from American Journal of Medicine, March 2005. www.ncbi.nlm.nih.gov/pubmed.

16   McCaughey, Betsey. "When Hospitals Become Killers." *The Wall Street Journal*, January 3, 2013.

17   "Nearly 60 percent of patients hospitalized for asthma are prescribed antibiotics." *CDDEP Weekly Digest*, July 29, 2016.

18   Sun, Lena H. "Hospital antibiotic use can put patients at risk, sudy says." *The Washington Post,* March 4, 2014.

19   Dall, Chris. "Fluoroquinolone stewardship may end at hospital door." *CIDRAP News*, February 13, 2019.

20   Park, Alice. "A Cautionary Tale About Antibiotics." *Time Magazine*, April 14, 2016.

21   Ranaivo, Yann. "UAB researchers: Inappropriate antibiotics use in ERs still a problem." *Birmingham Business Journal*, January 22, 2014.

22   McKay, Betsy. "New Push to Stop Overuse of Antibiotics in Nursing Homes." *The Wall Street Journal*, October 12, 2015.

23   Landro, Laura. "How Mainstream Medicine Is Stepping Out of the Mainstream." *The Wall Street Journal*, June 30, 2014.

24   Maeder, Thomas. *Adverse Events*, William Morrow and Company, Inc., New York NY, 1994, p. 405.

25 Schulte, Fred and Fry, Erika. "Electronic Health Records Creating a 'New Era' of Health Care Fraud, Officials Say." *Fortune*, December 23, 2019.

26 Evans, Melanie. "Tech Firms Get Identifiable Hospital Data." *The Wall Street Journal*, January 11, 2020.

27 Fried, Stephen. *Bitter Pills, Inside the Hazardous World of Legal Drugs*, Bantam Books, a division of Random House, May 1999, pp. 344-345.

28 Roe, Sam et al. "Filled without warning." *Chicago Tribune*, December 18, 2016.

29 Roe, Sam and Long, Ray. "Pharmacy chains improve drug alerts." *Chicago Tribune*, August 9, 2017.

30 Tomlinson, Kathy. "Pharmacists' failure to check drug risks leads to 'horrible' death." *CBC News*, October 6, 2014.

31 Hall, Colleen. "Senate Passes Bill to Prohibit Gag Clauses in Pharmacies." *Pharmacy Times*, September 18, 2018.

32 Martin, Philippe, PhD et al. "Effect of Pharmacist-Led Educational Intervention on Inappropriate Medication Prescriptions in Older Adults." *JAMA*, November 13, 2018.

33 Auta, Asa et al. "Global access to antibiotics without prescription in community pharmacies: a systematic review and meta-analysis." Journal of Infection, July 5, 2018.

34 Schwartz, Lisa M. and Woloshin, Steven. "The Drug Facts Box: Improving the communication of prescription drug information." Procedures of the National Academy of Science USA, August 20, 2013.

35 Eaton, Joe. "Black Market Meds Are Flooding the Nation's Pharmacies and Hospitals." *AARP Bulletin*, May 2016.

36 Fried, Stephen. *Bitter Pills*, p. 310.

37 Laliberte, Richard. "12 Ways the Heath Care System May Be Harming You." *AARP Bulletin*, September 2016.

38 Wolfe, Sidney M., MD. "Don't Get Sick in July." *Health Letter*, August 2010.

THE SITUATION WITH DOCTORS

*As to diseases, make a habit of two things—
to help, or at least, to do no harm.*

HIPPOCRATES

PHYSICIANS ARE OUR lifeline to good health and a long life. They spend years studying how to do that and then enter practice to share their knowledge with patients—caring, nurturing, prescribing, operating. They are overworked. They are burdened with information overload and increasing numbers of rules, regulations, and detailed recordkeeping. Doctors endure a multitude of pressures including persistent and pervasive marketing by pharmaceutical companies, in and out of their offices.

Our caregivers agree to do no harm when they take their oath of ethics. And yet it is disturbing how many do just that. It has been estimated that in the United States, 44,000 to 98,000 *deaths* per year may be attributed in some part to an inadvertent adverse effect or complication resulting from medical treatment or advice. These numbers were challenged more recently by a study reported in the *British Medical Journal* that estimates medical errors to account for

250,000 deaths and should be regarded as the third leading cause of death in the U.S., surpassed only by heart disease and cancer.[1] Even NASA's chief toxicologist got into the fray by calculating that medical error kills between 210,000 and 440,000 Americans each year.[2] Globally, medical errors harm as many as 40% of patients in primary and outpatient care, according to a 2019 report from the World Health Organization.[3]

Misdiagnosis, a frequent occurrence with fluoroquinolone toxicity, leads to permanent damage or death for more than 160,000 patients per year, according to researchers at Johns Hopkins University.[4] Injuries and disabilities from taking these drugs are more difficult to determine.

"In their practices," said the late Dr. Jay S. Cohen, author of a book about fluoroquinolones, "doctors often appear to blame other factors for damage done by the drugs Levaquin or Cipro. Unfortunately, many doctors do not know that fluoroquinolones can cause such severe, long-lasting reactions. When a reaction occurs, some doctors deny that it could have been caused by the drug. Doctors order a battery of tests to seek other causes, but the tests usually show nothing."[5]

Dr. Cohen's statement is confirmed by similar comments that are shared over and over by individuals harmed by taking these powerful antibiotics. There are hundreds of anguished anecdotes online of misdiagnosis and mistreatment that individuals have reported following the ingestion of fluoroquinolones.

I took my first and last pill. Within an hour I was layng [sic] on the bathroom floor listening to my boss calling my husband. I was obviously having an allergic reaction to the Levaquin. The left side of my face was swollen, my breathing was labored, I was chilled to the bone and shaking, nauseous and my heart was racing. I took a Benadryl, called the doctor and was assured that the worst would be over. It was just the beginning.

My health began to deteriorate immediately...I had a hysterectomy to get rid of the large fibroid tumors that appeared overnight. I had to leave my job and lay on the couch for a year as I suffered...abdominal cramping, headaches, shakiness, dizziness, loss of appetite and weight, nausea, hot and cold flashes, bouts of constipation and diarrhea, weakness, achiness, tinnitus, brain fog, sight problems, tremors, electrical zaps through my body, memory loss, heartburn, muscle wasting, strange rashes, back pain, tachycardia, fatigue, insomnia, joint and muscle pain, neuropathy, low blood pressure, food and chemical sensitivities, teeth breaking and more.

The doctors were able to find plenty of things wrong with me but nobody could put it together... Instead they found: gastritis, hiatal hernia, reflux, white matter lesions on my brain, hypothyroidism, thyroid autoimmune issues, lesions on my liver, granulomas in my spleen, kidney cysts, sclerosis in my spine and hip, reactive arthritis and finally... FLUOROQUINOLONE TOXICITY! ...I told every doctor that all I knew is that I'd been sick ever since an allergic reaction to Levaquin. And then I'd believe them when they said it couldn't be related. It wasn't until my mom had a friend pass away from taking a round of Levaquin and Cipro that we decided to look up the drug I had reacted to. Suddenly, everything I had gone through was there in so many stories![6]

Nine years floxed coming up on August 7th. I get angrier each year with the medical profession. They don't believe us.[7]

Physicians should be reporting all cases of adverse reactions suffered by their patients to the FDA's MedWatch, but as previously noted, rarely do. When 200 nurses were interviewed in Ohio, which has mandatory reporting laws, not one of them considered filing an adverse incident report with a state board or the FDA. "Why would I do that?" they often said. Even though most had filed from five to eight other types of incident reports internally sometime during their careers.[8]

ACCORDING TO DR. Jeffry A. Linder, writing in *JAMA Internal Medicine*, prescribing unnecessary antibiotics in primary care for acute respiratory infections is a common, inappropriate occurrence. They may be ordered because it is the easy option. Prescribers may perceive a want or explicit demand from a patient for an antibiotic or a desire to do something meaningful for the client. He or she may want to conclude a visit quickly or have an unrealistic fear of complications. Linder calls all of these reasons for providing unnecessary antibiotics *decision fatigue*.[9]

Physicians may honestly believe a patient's symptoms are "all in their head" if they are unable to find a diagnosis that fits the symptoms. They may blame the patient's personality instead of a pill.[10] Patients are sometimes tagged difficult, disruptive, borderline or treatment resistant. However, tagging patients with disrespectful and stigmatizing terminology could lead to improper diagnostic judgment with increased risk of a poor outcome.[11] Of course there are patients who are aggressive, demanding, and mean-spirited, and who imagine or invent symptoms. As many as 15% fall into this category.[12]

When patients present with their symptoms, doctors may refer to their Physician's Desk Reference (PDR). It lists symptoms, possible diseases or conditions, and suggests which drugs are preferred. It's an easy reference, but may not always be up to date on the hundreds of FDA-issued drug warnings. Instead, doctors may rely on pharmaceutical sales representatives who visit their offices frequently to keep them updated, at least on the drugs they happen to be selling. There are at least 10 other recommended data bases or apps in addition to the PDR that doctors can use today to make diagnoses, but it is unknown how many doctors actually use them.[13]

Fluoroquinolones are antibiotics. Antibiotics are not effective for treating viral infections, only bacterial diseases. Physicians often prescribe these medications, called the Big Guns, to patients without testing whether the infection is viral or bacterial. This results in overuse and, as we have seen, can unnecessarily cause serious adverse effects and injuries. These potent pills are called broad spectrum, meaning that they can be effective against a wide range of bacteria. They should be prescribed for serious, severe or life-threatening conditions, according to guidelines issued by the pharmaceutical companies as well as the FDA. The American Dental Association now recommends that doctors should not give prescriptions to patients for toothaches or dental work that does not involve fever or swollen lymph nodes.[14]

A rapid diagnostic test to determine whether an infection is viral or bacterial is readily accessible. It was approved by the FDA in 2017. Researchers found that the availability of this analysis doesn't reduce antibiotic prescribing, especially for lower respiratory tract infections. Even when the two-hour test is ordered, 57% of patients still receive antibiotics too early and 34% get a prescription for them in the hospital emergency room right away. Statistics were about the same for those who didn't have access to the test. Conclusion: Access to the test doesn't make a difference in prescribing habits.[15]

Even children are affected. *Journal Pediatrics* disclosed that when antibiotics are prescribed for youngsters, they are the Big Gun fluoroquinolones 50% of the time. And about 25% of those antibiotics were being prescribed for conditions for which they were ineffective or not approved. There are 30 to 40 million antibiotic orders written for children every year. Many are unnecessary or in error and result in a big win for Pharma and a significant risk for kids.[16]

Telemedicine is a relatively new medical practice. It involves diagnosing and prescribing by phone or through internet services without a doctor visit, and has become increasingly used by parents whose children are ill. The most common conditions parents contact these outside sources for are acute respiratory infections and those children are more likely to receive antibiotics. Parents are less likely to receive guided antibiotic management, such as dosage and how long to take them, compared to children visiting a doctor's office or urgent care facility.[17]

DESPITE DECADES OF increasing awareness of the potential for toxicity and the intensification of warnings by the FDA, fluoroquinolone prescribing patterns in the U.S. have remained largely unchanged. Of the 22 million fluoroquinolone orders written for patients, most are for a UTI. Prescriptions were most frequently written by primary practitioners but urologists were the largest contributing sub-specialty.

Urology Practice magazine cautions urologists about these drugs in this way: "It is essential that urologists remain up to date on fluoroquinolone toxicities and the related FDA warnings, which will help with timely recognition and subsequent discontinuation of this antibiotic."[18]

The over-prescribing of fluoroquinolones by physicians is pervasive. In the United States alone, doctors doled out some 32 million orders for these drugs several years ago. That made them the country's fourth-most popular antibiotic.[19]

The safety committee of the European Medicines Agency (EMA) recommends that treatments with fluoroquinolones be restricted and they should not be prescribed in the following situations:

- To treat self-resolving infections (such as throat infections).

- To prevent traveler's diarrhea or recurring lower urinary tract infections.

- To treat patients who have previously had serious adverse effects from a fluoroquinolone.

- To treat mild or moderately severe infections unless other antibacterial medicines commonly recommended for these infections cannot be used.[20]

To encourage physicians and other prescribers of drugs to rethink how they issue orders for antibiotics, the Agency for Healthcare Research and Quality (AHRQ) has developed a suggested safety program. The plan asks that prescribers use a Four-Moments framework.

Moment 1 asks: Does this patient have an infection that requires antibiotics? Prescribers should pause and consider if a noninfectious diagnosis is more likely.

Moment 2 asks: Have I ordered appropriate cultures before starting antibiotics? Lack of a culture can lead to unnecessary and prolonged antibiotic therapies.

Moment 3 asks: A day or more has passed. Can I stop antibiotics? Can I narrow therapy? Can I change from intravenous to oral therapy? Too often, the report suggested, a decision whether or not to continue antibiotic therapy is not revisited when more clinical and microbiological data become available.

Moment 4 asks: What duration of antibiotic therapy is needed for this patient's diagnosis? Traditionally, antibiotic prescribing practice has led to excessively long courses of treatment. Prescribers should support shorter durations of antibiotic therapy and advise according to each patient's health background and needs.

As for hospitalized patients, the AHRQ guidelines further suggest that a nurse or hospital pharmacist can prompt clinicians to actually write down plans for their patient's antibiotics. Doctors, medical practitioners and hospitalists should document every decision in the patient's progress notes that result from daily rounds and review treatment plans, including whether to continue antibiotic therapy, narrow it or switch to another medication.[21]

When it is necessary and acceptable to take these drugs, doctors rarely discuss with their patients the benefits *and* the risks *or* the conditions under which these medications should be taken. It's all in the pre-scription flyer at the pharmacy. One for fluoroquino-lones read: "Should not be taken at least two hours before or six hours after taking other products that may make it work less well, such as with supplements such as magnesium, calcium, antacids, calcium-en-riched juice, dairy products, yogurt, and more." Does the doctor tell you to avoid tanning booths and sun-lamps or to limit alcoholic beverages? Does he or she warn that children may be at greater risk taking these meds, or that if you are older you may be susceptible to tendon injuries?[22] Doctors' notes may include a protective disclaimer that these issues were discussed with the patient, even though they were not, as it was in my case.

INFORMED CONSENT AND shared decision-making are the new mantras for physicians. Getting doctors to a reasonable patient standard is the goal, but old habits are difficult to change. There is a practice known as "cookbook medicine" where a physician relies on a fixed approach to diagnosis that focuses on a patient's chief complaint and then rules out the worse-case scenarios. However, this can result in treating patients with a rigid, one-size-fits-all formula that may miss what is really going on.[23] In the case of fluoroquinolones, it has been shown that symptoms are wide-ranging and usually do not fit a pre-set diagnosis.

Unfortunately, care today may be determined by the corporate culture of a hospital, to which many doctors now belong in groups. Groups of physicians become employees, not independent doctors with their own businesses. It can influence the way they practice medicine. The physician-employee relationship can split a doctor's allegiance between his patient and who pays him. Hospital goals may not always coincide with a patient's best interests or the physician's best medical judgments.

In this new world, patients who are hospitalized are often seen not by their personal doctor but by the hospitalist. This hospital-employed physician or nurse practitioner likely never had contact with the patient previously. He or she provides little personal interaction or understanding of a patient's personal needs or extensive medical history.[24]

Sandrop Khurana, MBBS, wrote this in *The New Yorker* about the corporatization of medicine and fear of lawsuits:

"For the most part, healthcare institutions enforce a corporate-style model of productivity, which has turned health care providers into assembly-line workers under constant pressure to manage many patients in a limited amount of time in order to generate the most revenue possible. In addition, a fear of lawsuits compels physicians to see each medical decision and patient-care interaction through a legal filter. Physicians who are sued become hypervigilant and practice defensive medicine which costs more. Patients with headaches get CT scans to rule out tumors, and patients with viral infections are given antibiotics out of an abundance of caution."[25]

Treatment in the doctor's office has changed. Appointments are shorter and more abrupt, especially when doctors join groups owned by hospitals that insist upon efficiency and profits. Professionals are often focused on their computer screens instead of looking at patients directly to detect symptoms or listen carefully to complaints. Exams may be perfunctory. One doctor who never has a computer in the room when he's seeing his patients notes that having that device in the room is no different than when a patient is texting or talking on his phone while he is trying to make a diagnosis.[26]

TODAY, MANY PATIENTS will access the internet for medical information before or after a caregiver visit. They arrive with details or drug warnings that may or may not be familiar to their doctor. It should be a start to a productive discussion between patient and physician. However, it's an uneasy situation to challenge someone who has graduated from medical school with something that you have read on the internet.[27]

In recent years widespread access to websites and social media has reduced a physician's authority over medical information and given patients a window to a whole host of medical products and services. Internet-researching patients can alarm doctors as well as encourage dangerous decisions. Patients may mistakenly conclude they don't need a doctor. Individuals may also arrive at appointments with demands for expensive and unnecessary tests or drugs.

Direct-To-Consumer tests are readily available. Some testing that once required expensive equipment or an office or hospital visit can now be done at home. A patient can perform a do-it-yourself electrocardiogram on a $99 device that interfaces with a smartphone app. You can locate a wide array of lab tests that can easily be ordered and sent by mail. You can get complete blood cell counts, comprehensive metabolic panels, hepatitis C screening, and a variety of sexually transmitted disease screen panels on your own. Some tests are considered high quality while others don't meet the standards of clinical validity. There is also a burgeoning market for genetic testing that assesses consumers' risk of developing a large number of different diseases or conditions including late-onset Alzheimer's disease, Parkinson's disease, hereditary thrombophilia, or breast and ovarian cancer.

The smartphone has changed everything. You can now access a doctor through a service called Teledoc that allows you to get a physician on the phone within 15 minutes, handy if you have a medical emergency while driving, camping in a remote location, or if you live in a non-urban area. A doctor will provide immediate advice upon hearing your symptoms or direct you to the nearest hospital.

Tech companies are working toward making personal and hospital health records available to consumers through their computers and mobile devices. There are thousands of apps related to health or fitness available for smartphones, iPads or computers. Wearable devices such as smart watches and fitness devices are encouraging patient engagement in their personal health. They offer extensive data and education about hundreds of diseases, connections to health organizations, and more. Unanswered questions are whether these technological advances ultimately improve patient outcomes, lower costs or improve quality of life.[28]

All of this quick availability of medical information and health-related products and services allows patients to self-direct their own care. It's challenging for physicians who must manage a patient who has access to valid and non-valid medical information as well as the consequences of tests and screenings that they did not order. This new world of hi-tech medicine represents a radically altered balance of power between physician and patient.

Dr. Steven Joffe, writing in the *Journal of American Medicine*, suggests that in this new age of autonomy, physicians should learn to practice in three new ways: First, serve more as consultants or advisors. Second, continue to perform diagnostic and therapeutic procedures that patients are not able to carry out and make judgments about whether a given procedure is appropriate or not. Third, the doctor's function as gatekeeper with all the medical knowledge will have to change. Physicians will need to focus on follow-up services, such as immediate referral to a specialist when a patient learns that he or she is at risk of a certain disease.

Doctors should advocate for patient care that is driven by medical need rather than by patient demand. Patients will still depend upon their physicians for advice and diagnoses, but doctors will also be able to provide procedural expertise and access to restricted medical services.[29]

AS NOTED PREVIOUSLY, pharmaceutical companies spend millions of dollars to promote their drugs directly to physicians. Since August 2013, under The Sunshine Act, companies must record every promotional transaction they have with doctors and its cost, from pharma reps bearing pizza to industry compensation for advice on research, conference speaking engagements, travel, meals, royalties, stock, gifts and other payments in goods or services. At one time Pfizer alone paid doctors $194.5 million a year in gifts and compensations.

Patients can see what payments have been made to their doctors at the Centers for Medicare & Medicaid Services (https://openpaymentsdata.cms.gov/), which keeps tabs on those reports. Industry's failure to report fees and gifts generates penalties of at least $1,000 per transaction with the maximum annual fine capped at $1.14 million per company.[30] In 2020, the Sunshine Act will expand to include payments to physician assistants and advanced practical nurses.[31]

When ProPublica looked at payments to doctors by pharmaceutical and medical device companies, it was discovered that there were 700 physicians who had been paid more than $1 million each for giving promotional talks and consulting, aside from earning income from patient care. This didn't include money for doing research or receiving royalties from inventions.[32]

ProPublica analyzed records in several specialties and found that 74% of 150,000 physicians in one database received at least one industry payment in a specified year. The brand name prescribing rate was 10% for those who had not received payments and 30% for those who had received more than $5,000. Despite doctor denials, drug promotions and payments do work.

It is no accident that fluoroquinolones became blockbuster drugs. They have been marketed and promoted extensively to physicians as the best leading-edge antibiotics to combat infection. Doctors worldwide perceived them as miracle drugs. They prescribe them not only as powerful last resort remedies but for minor infections as well. This helped boost sales into the billions with soaring profits for pharmaceutical companies as well as corresponding increases in adverse events.

Direct-To-Consumer advertising impacts all drug use. Ask Your Doctor ads proliferate. When patients come to the doctor's office with requests for medications they have seen advertised, it puts a burden on doctors to educate patients on product claims, risks, benefits, medical need, and cost as they know it from reliable, or unreliable sources or from sales reps.[33] If they take the time to do that.

WHAT TO DO

- Don't ask for or demand an antibiotic from your doctor. Listen to his or her diagnosis and what is prescribed. The goal is to have a collaborative, non-threatening, relationship with your physician. If you show anger or are too critical, it can turn a physician or caregiver into a resister rather than a supporter.

- You can challenge your doctor's prescription and ask why it is necessary and why this drug is the best remedy. You have a right to refuse to take a medication if you feel it is prescribed only as a precaution or if you feel it is prescribed to protect the doctor and not you. It is recommended that new drugs not be taken for at least five years after they are on the market until safety is well-established.[34] You may ask your doctor if the drug being prescribed is at least five years old.

- You should always ask what are the risks of the medication being prescribed. If you feel the risks are too dangerous, discuss this with your doctor and ask if there are alternatives.

- You may ask if a lower dose of your medication would be just as effective.

- If you are asked to take a new medication, you can ask if other medications you are currently taking should then be discontinued. The fewer medications you take, the better. In addition, don't take a drug any longer than it is prescribed for.[35]

- You may ask a physician whether he or she is familiar with the severe adverse effects that occur with some patients after taking fluoroquinolones. If they are not, you can bring copies of information about this subject for them to your office visit or refer them to information found in this book or its Resources section.

- Assume that any symptoms you develop after starting a new drug, especially a fluoroquinolone, may be caused by that medication.

- Come to your doctor visit with a list of questions. Don't wait until later when your visit is about to end. You may get a hurried answer.[36]

- You can say no. You can say you would like to further research a medication or treatment on your own. You can get a second opinion. Your doctor should be amenable to your wishes. Remember, however, that he or she is making recommendations based upon his or her extensive medical experience and expert knowledge of your particular condition or disease.

- If there is an unknown individual in the room with you during your appointment, you have a right to ask who it is. If it is a sales rep, for example, you have a right to ask him or her to leave.

- Use trusted medical web sites when you do online research. The Mayo Clinic is one as is www.dailymed.nim.mih.gov. WebMD is another popular site. As part of shared decision-making, ask your doctor which websites he recommends for you.

- You can bring a cellphone photo or video to your doctor's office showing the beginnings of a rash or cough, for example, so that your provider can see progress or decline prior to your visit. You might take photos or videos of anything from accident scenes to epileptic seizures. These images could help your doctor make a correct diagnosis or recommend appropriate treatment. Provide copies to your physician so that he or she can add them to your health record.[37]

- Look around your doctor's office. Are there lots of notepads, pens, pencils, calendars, and posters that come from pharmaceutical companies? Although these are not major gifts, you can check whether your doctor has received payments or larger compensations from industry by accessing https://openpaymentsdata.cms.gov.

- If surgery or significant treatments are suggested, feel free to ask questions such as "Do I really need this surgery or treatment?" "What are the alternatives?" "What happens after surgery?" "Will I be given antibiotics in the hospital? If so, which ones and why?" You have the right to consider all options. If necessary, you can research your surgeon's "complication rate" at www.projectspropublica.org/surgeons.

• If tests are suggested, ask what they are and why they are needed. If it's "as a precaution," you have a right to refuse if you feel the test is unnecessary. Ask if there are alternatives.

• Your doctor deserves to hear about ALL of your symptoms and have a complete past history that may be affecting your health. Arrive at your appointment with a list of your current medications, dietary supplements, and recreational drug use. One overlooked pill or symptom may be critical for a correct diagnosis.

• You can ask your doctor what guidelines pertain to your condition. If you want to check them out yourself, you can look them up at the National Guideline Clearing House, www.guideline.gov.

• The doctor needs your help, too. It is your responsibility to take your medications as prescribed and to come to follow-up appointments when requested to do so.[38]

- And, finally, if you have been injured by taking a fluoroquinolone, ask your doctor to report it to the FDA's MedWatch site and then join an advocacy or support group. You'll find several in this book's Resources section.

Notes

1   Wilensky, Gail, PhD. "Changing Physician Behavior Is Harder Than We thought." *The JAMA Forum*, July 5, 2016.

2   Lieber, James B. "How to Make Hospitals Less Deadly." *The Wall Street Journal*, May 17, 2016.

3   Sutcliffe, Kathleen. "How to Reduce Medical Errors." *Time Magazine*, November 25, 2019.

4   Laura Landro. "The Biggest Mistake Doctors Make." *The Wall Street Journal*, November 17, 2013.

5   www.fatsn.org. "The Cure That Kills" by Stan Cox, January 2008.

6   www.floxiehope.com/ keris-recovery-story-levaquin-toxicity

7   Bequealth, Janet. www.facebook.com/longtimefloxed, July 24, 2019.

8   www.patientsafety.com

9   Linder, Jeffrey A., MD, MPH et al. "Time of Day and the Decision to Prescribe Medicines." *JAMA Internal Medicine*, October 6, 2014.

10   Fried, Stephen. *Bitter Pills, Inside the Hazardous World of Legal Drugs*, Bantam Books, a division of Random House, May 1999, p. 26.

11   Michelle, Joy, MD et al. "The Ethics of Behavioral Health Information Technology." *JAMA*, September 8, 2016.

12   Reddy, Sumathi. "When Patients Are a Pain for Their Doctors." *The Wall Street Journal*, April 4, 2016.

13   Whalen, Jeanne. "Health-Care Apps That Doctors Use." *The Wall Street Journal*, November 17, 2013.

14   "New ADA guideline recommends against using antibiotics for toothaches." *CDDEP Weekly Digest*, November 4, 2019.

15   "Diagnostic test does not reduce antibiotic prescribing."
     CDDEP Weekly Digest, June 7, 2018.

16   Reddy, Sumathi. "Antibiotics Do's and Don'ts." *The Wall
     Street Journal*, August 20, 2013.

17   Ray, Kristin N. et al. "Antibiotic Prescribing During Pediatric
     Direct-to-Consumer Telemedicine Visits." *Pediatrics*, April 2019.

18   Averch, Timothy D. "Fluoroquinolones: The Emergence of
     Toxicity Syndrome." *Urology Practice*, September 2017.

19   Marchant, Jo. "When antibiotics turn toxic." *Nature*,
     March 21, 2018.

20   MacVane, Shawn, PHARMD. "Fluoroquinolone
     Antibiotics: More Recommendations for Prudent
     Use." *ContagionLive*, October 29, 2018.

21   Tamma, Pranita D., MD, MHS et al. "Rethinking How
     Antibiotics Are Prescribed." www.jamanetwork.com,
     December 27, 2018.

22   "Levofloxacin and Ciprofloxacin." Medication reports
     provided by Rite Aid Pharmacy, August 10, 2018.

23   Landro, Laura. "When Doctors Don't Listen: How to
     Avoid Misdiagnoses and Unnecessary Tests." *The
     Wall Street Journal*, February 19, 2013.

24   Zinberg, Joel, MD. "Physicians who are employees of
     hospitals will split their allegiances between their
     employers and patients." *The Wall Street Journal*,
     December, 22, 2014.

25   Khurana, Sandeep, MBBS. "The Mail." *The New Yorker,*
     June 29, 2015.

26   "The Doctor Will See You (Or Her Screen) Now." *The
     Wall Street Journal*, May 15, 2016.

27   Baumann, Nick. "My Big Levaquin Adventure."
     Mother Jones, December 7, 2010.

28   Dameff, Christian, MD et al. "Personal Health Records.
      More Promising in the Smartphone Era?" www.
      jamanetwork.com, January 11, 2019.

29   Joffe, Steven, MD, MPH. "The New Age of Patient
      Autonomy." www.jamanetwork.com, October 16, 2018.

30   Loftus, Peter. "Doctors Face New Scrutiny Over Gifts;
      New Health Law Calls for Increased Disclosures." *The
      Wall Street Journal*, August 22, 2013.

31   Ortiz, Selena E., MPH and Rosenthal, Meredith B., PhD.
      "Medical Marketing, Trust, and the Patient-Physician
      Relationship." *JAMA*, January 8, 2019.

32   Ornstein, Charles et al. "We Found Over 700 Doctors
      Who Were Paid More than a Million Dollars by Drug and
      Medical Device Companies." www.propublica.org, October
      17, 2019.

33   Ortiz, Selena E., MPH and Rosenthal, Meredith B., PhD.
      "Medical Marketing, Trust, and the Patient-Physician
      Relationship." *JAMA*, January 8, 2019.

34   Light, Donald W. "New Prescription Drugs: A Major
      Health Risk with Few Offsetting Advantages." www.ethics.
      harvard.edu/blog.

35   "Ten Rules for Safer Drug Use." *Worst Pills Best Pills, A
      Consumer's Guide to Avoiding Drug-Induced Death or Illness.*
      Pocket Books, a division of Simon & Schuster, Inc., New
      York NY, 1990, pp. 864-869.

36   Paturel, Amy. "How to talk so your doctor will listen."
      AARP Bulletin, January-February 2017.

37   Gribben, Valerie. "Valerie Gribben: Take Two Photos and
      Call Me in the Morning." *The Wall Street Journal*, August
      12, 2013.

38   Laliberte, Richard. "12 Ways the Heath Care System May
      Be Harming You." *AARP Bulletin*, September 2016.

EPILOGUE

CHANGE IS COMING. We can hope.

ADVOCACY GROUPS IN the fluoroquinolone support community are finally beginning to be heard, although still minimally. Testimony given by officers of the Quinolone Vigilance Foundation (QVF) before the FDA a few years ago resulted in a new black box warning. This nonprofit organization raises awareness about fluoroquinolones and their dangers and provides funds for research on toxicity.

Public Citizen has been an advocate for the safety of fluoroquinolones for years, sending out news releases, testifying before congressional committees, and urging the FDA to be fair and honest in its approvals of drugs. This diligent group has revealed misdemeanors as well as major wrong doings in the pharmaceutical industry, spotlighted questionable practices in the medical field, and identified various shortcomings at the FDA. It's an important monitor of public health in the U.S.

A Fluoroquinolone Awareness Conference was held in November 2019 in Ottawa, Canada. It was initiated by a group of victims, scientists and researchers belonging to an organization called the Fluoroquinolone Research and Discussion Group. This first-of-its-kind conference featured noted scientists, informed speakers and victims. The purpose was to create more awareness about the drug's disabling injuries and urge change in policy and usage.

As recently as October 2018, the European Medicines Agency (EMA) recommended that *all fluoroquinolone antibiotics be removed from the market.* Its Pharmacovigilance Risk Assessment Committee made this stark determination after interviewing patients, healthcare professionals and academics. The announcement advised that use of fluoroquinolones should be restricted from taking by mouth, injection or inhalation.

Stewardship, especially in hospitals, seems to be making some progress. Restrained use of antibiotics, including fluoroquinolones, is beginning to be recognized by selected hospital systems and new rules hopefully implemented.

Several years ago, the FDA asked twenty-six pharmaceutical companies to voluntarily phase out using antibiotics for promoting growth in animals that would be processed for meat or revise how these drugs should be used. All but one company agreed. This voluntary process did not require that companies limit antibiotic drugs for disease prevention when animals were held in crowded conditions such as at factory farms. Usage continued.

Growth hormones and antibiotics to prevent disease are commonly given to animals raised for food. These drugs then make their way to our tables as meat and we ingest them. What these common industry practices do is to promote antibiotic overuse and drug resistance in animals as well as humans.

At the end of 2018, major food companies agreed to improve antibiotic stewardship in animal production. Food companies, livestock producers and agricultural associations agreed to commit to transparency, consistency and accountability in their use of antibiotics. Significant companies and trade associations agreed, including McDonald's, Tyson Foods and the National Pork Producers Council. This showed progress; however, companies did not agree to *eliminate* giving these drugs to their farm animals.

The coronavirus pandemic will change healthcare. Telemedicine will surge as both patients and doctors develop new relationships online and with virtual visits. In the new normal, perhaps doctors will return to more personal and compassionate care for patients and listen to them more carefully. Complaints of adverse events occurring after taking fluoroquinolones, we can hope, will be taken seriously and listened to. In addition, let us hope that habits of kindness and altruistic purpose will endure and infect the entire medical community, forcing even Big Pharma to devote more resources to developing safe drugs rather than promoting big profits.

A few new promising antibiotics for attacking bacteria are in the drug development pipeline. They are being fast-tracked by the FDA to try to combat the rising tide of antibiotic resistance around the world. New antibiotics called malacidins and arylomycins hope to address this fearful issue by building cell walls against infection or targeting negative bacteria. Let's hope that new antibiotics will be thoroughly tested for dangerous adverse reactions prior to approval so that the heartbreaking stories of fluoroquinolone-caused injuries will not be repeated.

Media coverage of fluoroquinolone issues has been surprisingly consistent and extensive for years and years. *(See Bibliography.)* Even so, immense and continuing media coverage of the harms caused by these medications hasn't seemed to make much of a dent. There hasn't been major change in drug safety approval. Fluoroquinolones have continued to be sold without effective monitoring. Rarely have these antibiotics been discontinued because of harm and injury.

In December 2017, J&J quietly took Levaquin off the market. The formula survives, however, in thousands of generics, pills still taken by consumers every day. Branded Cipro and Avelox continue to be manufactured and sold by Bayer in large quantities worldwide.

Research indicates that fluoroquinolones may be making changes to our DNA. These antibiotics can actually change the structure of our cells. If this can be proven without a doubt, the risks of taking these medications should raise loud alarms and calls for immediate action in the medical and pharmaceutical communities as well as with federal regulators. ***Changing your DNA with drugs without your permission is immoral and invasive beyond description.***

There are critical questions that require immediate research and clinical testing to ensure safe ingestion of fluoroquinolones:

- Why do some patients endure severe reactions?

- Why do some patients have only a mild reaction?

- Why do some patients have only one adverse event and others have multiple injuries?

- Why do most patients have no reactions whatsoever?

- Why do some patients have immediate reactions while others have ongoing or recurring events weeks, months, or even years later?

- Why do some patients recover while others do not?

- Why do patients suffer with so many different reactions: some have hallucinations, tinnitus or vision problems, while others have torn tendons, nerve damage or severe anxiety?

It is simply amazing that with all the information about fluoroquinolones available in books, newspapers, magazine articles, on television, stories by the hundreds on the internet, and dozens of flourishing support groups, plus warnings and label changes by the FDA issued for more than 40 years, there has not been significant change in the safe use and prescribing of these drugs. It is unconscionable that these antibiotics are still on the market and have not been modified or tightly restricted.

A new fluoroquinolone was recently approved by the FDA. It's for treating ear infections in children. This potent class of drugs that has been shown to have created holes in young eardrums and has harmed so many others for so many years has now been approved and recommended for use in infants ...*as young as six months old*.

We can do better than this.

RESOURCES

BOOKS

Adverse Reactions by Thomas Maeder. William Morrow and Company, Inc., New York, NY. 1994.

This is the story of the first broad spectrum antibiotic to be chemically created and its miracle cures along with its tragic adverse effects. It is a fascinating history of the powerful drug chloramphenicol. Maeder discusses in detail how this first blockbuster antibiotic impacted the pharmaceutical industry and regulation in negative ways, ways that continue even today. This book questions the ethics and economics of the modern drug industry and ongoing controversies.

Bad Pharma, How Drug Companies Mislead Doctors and Harm Patients by Ben Goldacre, Faber and Faber, Inc., New York, NY. 2012.

Goldacre, physician and "Bad Science" columnist for the Guardian, argues that the influence of drug companies systematically corrupts the way medical knowledge is gathered and disseminated. He attacks non-evidence based clinical trials, biased publication practices, nefarious industry marketing and dishonest regulation procedures.

Bitter Pills, Inside the Hazardous World of Legal Drugs. By Stephen Fried. Random House, Inc., New York, NY. 1998.

The writer's wife, Diane, was prescribed a forerunner of today's fluoroquinolone pills and suffered life-changing adverse effects. The devastating experience caused Fried to write this well-researched book of investigative reporting as he tried to find answers about how and why this could happen.

Deadly Medicines and Organised Crime. By Peter C. Gotzsche. Radcliffe Publishing, Ltd., London, UK. 2013.

This is a powerful book by a noted British physician who worked with clinical trials and regulatory affairs in the drug industry and co-founded The Cochrane Collaboration, internationally recognized as the benchmark for high-quality information about the effectiveness of health care. The book is a shocker, revealing inside information about what "crimes and misdemeanors" are happening in the pharmaceutical industry and the broader medical world and how we have become the victims.

Deadly Monopolies by Harriet A. Washington. Random House, Inc., New York, NY. 2012.

A disturbing book that details the monopolistic patents of genes, questionable drugs, and the corporate control of medical practice and its harmful, even lethal, consequences for public health.

Our Daily Meds by Melody Petersen. Picador, New York, NY. 2009

An eye-opening, chilling account of the incredibly pervasive and corrupt influence of the pharmaceutical industry in America, as told by a journalist who wrote for years about the pharmaceutical industry at The New York Times. Petersen connects the dots to show how subtle, far-reaching and dangerous Big Pharma's powers have become.

PHARMA, Greed, Lies, and the Poisoning of America by Gerald Posner. Avid Reader Press, Simon & Shuster, New York, NY, 2020.

An impressive, well-researched book by an award-winning journalist that traces drug industry history and details the first mega drug marketing campaign. That multi-million-dollar crusade brought huge profits to Pfizer for one of the first antibiotics, Terramycin. Its innovative sales strategy became an industry model for generating enormous profits regardless of ethics or safety. The marketing genius of Arthur Sackler, who rolled out that first sales campaign, and his secretive and vastly-profitable family drug company and publishing enterprises are the subject of much of this book as well as the family's irresponsible promotion of opioids to blockbuster status.

Pharmageddon by David Healy. University of California Press, Berkeley and Los Angeles, CA. 2012.

Written by a psychiatrist and scientist, this book meticulously documents developments in the medical-industrial complex as well as pharmaceutical companies' creation of blockbuster drugs that require them to overhype benefits and deny real hazards.

Poison Pills, the Untold Story of the Vioxx Drug Scandal by Tom Nesi, St. Martin's Press, New York, NY. 2008.

The title tells it all, the tale of how far a drug maker went to bury safety information about its powerful new drug because it might hurt sales only to see it cause harm and death to more than 100,000 unsuspecting patients.

Protecting America's Health by Philip J. Hilts. The University of North Carolina Press, Chapel Hill and London. 2003.

This book presents the grand sweep of one hundred years of drug regulation in the U.S. It is fascinating coverage of historically significant events including stories about the laws and government regulations of the prescription drug business from 1903-2003 and their implications on health care.

The Hidden Dangers of Antibiotics. By Jay S. Cohen, MD. Square One Publishers, Garden City Park, NY. 2018.

Written by a nationally recognized expert on prescription drugs, this book spotlights the hazards that this physician saw when his patients took Cipro, Levaquin and other fluoroquinolone antibiotics. He focuses on exposing the destructive capability of these particular drugs and their far-reaching harm, providing guidance on dealing with the consequences, and advocating for awareness and change. Dr. Cohen published an earlier book in 2015 called How We Can Halt The Cipro & Levaquin Catastrophe: The Worst Medication Disaster in U.S. History. This book is out of print. Only very expensive used copies are available on amazon.com.

The Risks of Prescription Drugs by Donald W. Light. Columbia University Press, New York, NY. 2010.
Professor Light discusses critical questions such as how the burden of prescription risk has shifted from Big Pharma to individuals, how the FDA provides inadequate protection from unsafe drugs, and how medicine has become commercialized. Access his fact-filled blog at www.pharmamyths.net.

Worst Pills Best Pills, A Consumer's Guide to Avoiding Drug-Induced Death or Illness. Simon & Shuster, Inc., New York, NY. 2005.
Compiled by nine leading physicians and pharmacists and the Public Citizen's Health Research Group, this invaluable guide analyzes more than 500 drugs and designates close to 200 medications that should not be taken at all. A large volume, this directory recommends

drug alternatives as well as a list of "10 Rules for Safer Drug Use."

SUPPORT AND ADVOCACY GROUPS

Fluoroquinolone Antibiotic Toxicity Syndrome Network (FATSN). A nonprofit organization founded "by individuals whose lives have been forever interrupted and changed by severe adverse reactions to Fluoroquinolone Antibiotics: Avelox, Cipro, Levaquin, Floxin." An international community that strives to spread awareness globally through education, advocacy and community support. www.fatsn.org.

Fluoroquinolone Research and Discussion Group. This online closed group seeks to share peer-reviewed legitimate research and articles about fluoroquinolone side effects. It posts current media reports and encourages victims to share their stories. The organization holds an annual FQ Rally in Toronto, celebrates a FQ Friday, and plans international conferences to increase awareness, report on research and hear stories. www.facebook. com/fluoroquinoloneresearchanddiscussiongroup.

Public Citizen. An independent organization that advocates for safer, more effective drugs, medical devices and other products as well as physician accountability, and spotlights issues with Big Pharma. Staff testify in Washington on health issues and support important medical legislation. It monitors the Recall Unsafe Drugs Act of 2017 introduced in February, 2017. Its Health Research Group was founded in 1971 by Sidney Wolfe, MD and Ralph Nader and produces a monthly *Health Newsletter* as well as forefront information for patients at www.worstpills.org. Public Citizen website: www.citizen.org.

Quinolone Vigilance Foundation. The mission of this nonprofit charitable organization is to build an international awareness movement by advocating for patients harmed by fluoroquinolone antibiotics, educating medical professionals, strengthening warning labels, reducing antibiotic resistance through the vigilant use of antibiotics, and funding research on fluoroquinolone toxicity. www.saferpills.org.

WEB SITES

www.askapatient.com. Go to this website and type in the name of your medication to see comments by those who may have had a medical reaction to your drug.

www.ciproispoison.com. This is an angry yet reasoned account of the devastating experience one formerly healthy and active young person had after taking Cipro and the untold information he uncovered about fluoroquinolones. His story of a life ruined is not uncommon. This website was established, he says, "as the warning I wish I had been given."

www.fda.gov/Safety/MedWatch/. This is where you will find the FDA's MedWatch online form for reporting adverse effects from taking fluoroquinolones.

www.floxiehope.com. Locate information and resources here for individuals who have been "floxed" by fluoroquinolones. Numerous posts from victims as well as media stories, links and resources.

www.fqwallofpain.com. Hundreds of victims of fluoroquinolones have posted their photos and heartbreaking stories of severe reactions and disabling conditions they experienced including many disbelieving responses from doctors, nurses, and ER personnel. Postings began in 2014.

www.fqresearch.org. Site dedicated to presenting research, information and warnings about fluoroquinolone toxicity in order to prevent further harm. Research articles are posted about adverse events and health issues. Link to "Certain Adverse Effects," a six-part movie about fluoroquinolones.

www.fqvictims.org. Resource of victim stories, articles on fluoroquinolone issues, link to MedWatch, news stories, resources and advocacy.

www.levaquinadversesideeffect.com. "Hurt by Levaquin" site created by John Fratti includes extensive information about his long-term debilitating experience, details about the drug and its manufacturer, media coverage, medical references, links and advocacy. Archives extend back to 2008.

www.medicationssense.com. Site established by the late Dr. Jay S. Cohen, a drug expert, to help patients and their doctors make informed, intelligent choices about medications to maximize benefits and minimize risk. Includes a list of books and thoughtful articles about Levaquin, Cipro and Avelox and details of his advocacy efforts nationwide on behalf of fluoroquinolone-affected patients.

www.myquinstory.info. Extensive information shared to enlighten the public on fluoroquinolones and enable informed drug choices. Includes a multitude of articles and opinion pieces. Valuable links. Created by a fluoroquinolone victim.

www.nabp.net. Site of the National Association of Boards of Pharmacy lists accredited online pharmacies under Programs and VIPPS.

www.openpaymentsdata.cms.gov. Find out if your doctor or teaching hospital has accepted payments from industry and if so, how much and for what.

www.perilouspills.com. A blog on this site shares current news about fluoroquinolones and issues that affect use of these antibiotics as well as a place where victims can tell their stories.

www.youtube.com. "The Dangers of

Fluoroquinolones." October 2081. Victim Jonathan Furman speaks about his long-term toxicity and the research he has uncovered. (Numerous other fluoroquinolone videos can be found on YouTube.)

FACEBOOK GROUPS

There are many open and closed fluoroquinolone groups on www.facebook.com. Each site hosts from several hundred to more than ten thousand members.

Cipro Ciprofloxacin Toxicity Group
Floxed Activists Unite
Floxed Documentary Outreach
Floxed Ladies Only
Floxie Farm Group
Floxie Finder
Floxie Hangout
Floxies Uncensored
Fluoroquinolone Assistance Group
Fluoroquinolone Files Library
Fluoroquinolone Induced Endocrine Problems
Fluoroquinolone Induced Gastrointestinal Problems
Fluoroquinolone Induced Mitochondrial
Disfunction and DNA Damage
Fluoroquinolone Induced Musculoskeletal Group
Fluoroquinolone Induced Vision Damages Group
Fluoroquinolone Toxicity Group Solutions
Fluoroquinolone Twilight Zone
Fluoroquinolone Victim Assistance Group
FQ Food and Beverage

FQ Survivors Marketplace
FQAD Fluoroquinolone-Associated Disability
Public Group
FQAD Induced Metabolic Disruption
FQs Europe-Fluoroquinolone-Toxicity
FQT Live Chat
Hacking Fluoroquinolones
Iodines for Fluoroquinolone Toxicity
Life With Severe Fluoroquinolone Toxicity
Syndrome
Long Time Floxed
Natural Healing for Floxies
Stem Cell Recovery for Fluoroquinolone Toxicity
24/7
Surviving Antibiotic Adverse Reactions Avelox,
Cipro, Levaquin, Floxin
Vaccines in the Realm of FQ Toxicity

SELECTED BIBLIOGRAPHY

Code Key:
AARP: American Association of Retired Persons
CDDEP: Center for Disease Dynamics, Economics and Policy
CDER: Center For Drug Evaluation and Research
CIDRAP: Center for Infectious Disease Research and Policy
CMAJ: Canadian Medical Association Journal
JAMA: Journal of the American Medical Association
QVF: Quinolone Vigilance Foundation

"9 Types of Medication Older Adults Should Use With Caution." www.aarp.org, July 19, 2011.

"21st Century Cures: Gift to Big Pharma, Bad Deal for Patients." *Worst Pills Best Pills Newsletter*, February 2017.

"30% of antibiotics prescribed in hospitals are unnecessary." *PBS NewsHour*, August 3, 2017.

"A Brief Guide to Understanding Medical Studies." *Worst Pills Best Pills Newsletter*, September 2014.

"A Call for Innovation in Drug Regulation." *The Wall Street Journal*, February 26, 2013.

"A Closer Look at 'Needless' Hospital Deaths." *The Wall Street Journal*, May 23, 2016.

"A Dangerous Gap in FDA Recall Authority." *Worst Pills Best Pills Newsletter*, September 2014.

"A Guide to Drug Safety Terms at the FDA." Consumer Health Information, www.fda.gov.

"A Guide to Drugs for Uncomplicated Urinary Tract Infections." *Worst Pills Best Pills Newsletter,* May 2016.

"A Healthy Dose of Skepticism Is Well Justified." *Worst Pills Best Pills Newsletter,* November 2012.

"A Large Outbreak of Clostridium Difficile-Associated Disease With An Unexpected Proportion of Deaths and Colectomies at a Teaching Hospital Following Increased Fluoroquinolones Use." *Infection Control and Hospital Epidemiology,* March, 2005.

"Accentuate the Positive, Eliminate the Negative." *Worst Pills Best Pills Newsletter,* May 2013.

"Adverse Drug Reactions: How Serious Is the Problem and How Often and Why Does It Occur?" *Worst Pills Best Pills Newsletter,* November 2010.

"Adverse side effects send about 4.5 million Americans to the doctor's office or emergency room each year." *AARP Bulletin,* September 2, 2011.

"Alternatives to Fluoroquinolones." www.jamanetwork. com, October 4, 2016.

"An association found between childhood antibiotic treatment and later development of IBD (Inflammatory Bowel Disease)." *Journal of Pediatrics,* October 2012.

"An Uncontrollable Outbreak." *The New York Times,* editorial, August 29, 2012.

"Anthrax and Cipro." pfpc@istar.ca, Parents of Fluoride Poisoned Children (PFPC), Vancouver BC, Canada, reprint in *Wellness Directory of Minnesota*.

"Antibiotic Misuse: Dangerous for Everyone." *Worst Pills, Best Pills Newsletter*, July, 2016.

"Antibiotic overuse varies across U.S." *Chicago Tribune*, November 16, 2012.

"Antibiotic prescriptions for urinary tract infections are all too common in hospitals and nursing homes." *Weekly Digest*, CDDEP, October 21, 2016.

"Antibiotic resistance developing more rapidly." *Weekly Digest*, CDDEP, April 11, 2014.

"Antibiotic stewardship efforts may be paying off: antibiotic prescribing and spending in U.S. is declining." *Weekly Digest*, CDDEP, September 3, 2017.

"Antibiotic Use Aids MRSA Spread in Hospital and Infection Control Measures Do Little to Prevent It, Says Hospital Study." *ScienceDaily*, September 20, 2012.

"Antibiotic use linked to Type 2 diabetes." *Weekly Digest*, CDDEP, September 4, 2015.

"Antibiotics may accelerate bacterial reproduction." *Weekly Digest*, CDDEP, February 3, 2017.

"Antibiotics to Avoid Like the Plague Due to FDA's Oversight Failure." www.mercola.com.

"Antibiotics, Common Heartburn Drugs and Spread of Potentially Fatal Intestinal Infection." *Worst Pills Best Pills*, August 2015.

"Antimicrobial resistance 'future global health crisis' reports Canada's Public Health Officer." CMA releases new policy on AMR." *Canadian Medical Association*, www.cma.ca, June 16, 2019.

"Assessing FDA Performance: Approval Speed Is Not the Answer." *Worst Pills, Best Pills Newsletter,* July 2014.

"Battling the superbugs." *Chicago Tribune*, editorial, June 4, 2016.

"Big Pharma's Self-Promoting Media Campaign." *Worst Pills Best Pills Newsletter,* April 2017.

"Bitter Pill." www.globalnews.ca, March 14, 2012.

"Brain-injured John Fratti meets with the FDA over Levaquin." *PRNewswire*, August 6, 2010.

"Carey & Danis LLC Announces Four Lawsuits against the Makers of Levaquin." *Business Wire*, September 3, 2009.

"Certain Antibiotics Spur Widening Reports of Severe Side Effects." *PBS NewsHour*, June 16, 2011.

"Ciprofloxacin has dramatic effects on the mitochondrial genome: Antibiotics should be used cautiously." *ScienceDaily*, October 8, 2018.

"Ciprofloxacin Otic Suspension (Otiprio) for Acute Otitis Externa." *JAMA*, October 2, 2018.

"Ciprofloxacin side effects ranged up to 19% in postal workers." *CIDRAP News*, November 30, 2001.

"Clinical trials, For my next trick…" *The Economist*, March 26, 2016.

"Common and Rare Side Effects for Levaquin Oral." www.webmd.com.

"Confessions of a Representative of the Pharmaceutical

Industry." www.youtube.com.

"Consumer Wins Levaqin Lawsuit." www.aboutlawsuits. com, December 10, 2010.

"Curbing the Overuse of Antibiotics." *The Kojo Nnamdi Show*, *WAMU*, American University, Washington, DC, February 19, 2014.

"Dangerously Blind Faith in Drug Advertising and the FDA Drug-Approval Process." *Worst Pills Best Pills Newsletter*, November 2011.

"Diagnostic test does not reduce antibiotic prescribing." *Weekly Digest*, CDDEP, June 7, 2018.

"Doctors Accepting Bribes, Betraying Patients." *Worst Pills Best Pills Newsletter*, August, 2016.

"Doctors push drugmakers' line as conflicts abound." *Portland Press Herald*, editorial, December 28, 2016.

"Does $760m a Year of Industry Funding Affect the FDA's Drug Approval Process?" *Worst Pills, Best Pills Newsletter*, February, 2015; reprint from *British Medical Journal*, August 5, 2014.

"DRIVE-AB CONFERENCE 2016: Stimulating innovation, sustainable use of global access to antibiotics." *Weekly Digest*, CDDEP, May28, 2016.

"Drug Companies Eager to Market and Sell to Older Adults but Not To Adequately Test Them." *Worst Pills Best Pills Newsletter*, May 2012.

"Drug Company CEOs: Rewarded For Illegal Acts?" *Worst Pills Best Pills Newsletter*, August 2013.

"Drug Industry's Unacceptable Delays in Reporting Adverse Events to the FDA." *Worst Pills, Best Pills*

Newsletter, November 2015.

"Drug maker halts production of antibiotic Levaquin with reported side effects but risk remains." *WFTS,* Tampa Bay, FL, October 9, 2018.

"Drug maker stopped making popular antibiotic Levaquin amid concerns about mental health side effects." *RTV6,* Tampa Bay, FL, July 17, 2018.

"Drugs & Medications-levaquin side effects." www. webmd.com.

"Drugs@FDA: FDA Approved Drug Products." www. accessdata.fda.gov.

"Escalating Criminal and Civil Violations: Pharma Has Corporate Integrity? Not Really." *Worst Pills Best Pills Newsletter,* March, 2014.

"F.D.A. Creeps Forward." *New York Times,* editorial, January 11, 2012.

"FAERS Reporting by Patient Outcomes by Year." www.fda.gov/Drugs/ GuidanceComplianceRegulatoryInformation.

"FDA Approves New Indication for Levaquin Tablets/ Injection." *PR Newswire,* September 14, 2000.

"FDA approves safety labeling changes for fluoroquinolones." www.fda.gov.

"FDA Drug Safety Communication: FDA advises restricting fluoroquinolone antibiotic use for certain uncomplicated infections; warns about disabling side effects that can occur together." www.fda.gov, May 12, 2016.

"FDA Drug Safety Communication: FDA requires label

changes to warn of risk for possibly permanent nerve damage from antibacterial fluroquinolone drugs taken by mouth or by injection." www.fda.gov, August 22, 2013.

"FDA Extends Marketing Exclusivity for LEVAQUIN." *PR Newswire*, March 14, 2007.

"FDA Finally Changes Warning Label." *Newsletter for Summer*, QVF, *2016*, July 31, 2016.

"FDA Joins Hands With Industry to Weaken Its Own Rules." *Worst Pills Best Pills Newsletter*, February 2016.

"FDA Requires Safety Label Changes for Fluoroquinolones." *HealthDay News*, July 11, 2018.

"FDA Requires Stronger Warnings for Commonly Used Antibiotics." *Worst Pills, Best Pills Newsletter*, February 2017.

"FDA warns side effects may outweigh antibiotic's benefits." *Portland Press Herald*, May 14, 2016.

"Fluoroquinolone and quinolone antibiotics: PRAC recommends new restrictions on use following review of disabling and potentially long-lasting side effects." www.ema.Europa.eu, The European Medicines Agency, October 16, 2018.

"Fluoroquinolone Antibiotics Associated with Increased Risk of Retinal Detachment." *Worst Pills Best Pills Newsletter*, July 2012.

"Fluoroquinolones Linked to Life-Threatening Blood Vessel Complications." *Worst Pills Best Pills Newsletter*, April 2016.

"Hillary Clinton and Levaquin, A Teachable Moment." www.myquinstory.info, September 16, 2016.

"Hospitals Band Together to Bypass Big Pharma, Start Their Own Drug Company." *Worst Pills Best Pills Newsletter*, November 2018.

"How can we find out if our doctors have taken money from industry?" *Worst Pills Best Pills Newsletter*, October, 2016.

"How Many Pills Do Your Elderly Patients Take Each Day? *HCPLive*, Healthcare Professionals Network, October 4, 2010.

"How should we approach our doctors about a medicine that *Worst Pills, Best Pills News* designates as Do Not Use or Do Not Use for Seven Years?" *Worst Pills, Best Pills Newsletter*, September 2016.

"Human consumption of antibiotics up 65% in fifteen years." *Weekly Digest*, CDDEP, April 11, 2018.

"Human microbiota a promising source for future antibiotics, *Weekly Digest*, CDDEP, July 29, 2016.

"Hurt By Levaquin." www.levaquinadversesideeffects.com.

"Inadvertent Adverse Reactions With Commonly Used Drugs." *Worst Pills Best Pills Newsletter*, January 2012.

"Industry Money Undermines the Doctor-Patient Relationship." *Worst Pills, Best Pills Newsletter*, June 2016.

"Initial Ruling in Industry Lawsuit Threatens FDA's Regulation of Drugs." *Worst Pills, Best Pills*, October 2015.

"Is it safe for general practices to prescribe fewer antibiotics?" *Weekly Digest*, CDDEP, July 9, 2016.

"Is your Prescription Medication Safe?" www.globalnews. ca, March 15, 2012.

"LEVAQUIN 500MG TABLETS. INGREDIENT NAME: LEVOFLOXACIN." Drug information, Walgreen Pharmacy, Northbrook, IL, May 17, 2012.

"Levaquin Approved to Treat or Prevent Plague." *U.S. News & World Report*, April 2012.

"Levaquin is the Preferred Quinolone Among More Than Half of All General Medical-Surgical Hospitals in the United States." *PR Newswire*, December 2, 2008.

"Levofloxacin. Important Warning:" *MedlinePlus*, National Institutes of Health (NIH), October 15, 2016.

"Levofloxacin: MedlinePlus Drug Information." www. medlineplus.gov.

"List of largest pharmaceutical companies by revenue." www.wikipedia.com.

"Little-known dangers of fluoroquinolones." *Weekly Digest*, CDDEP, April 11, 2018.

"Medical errors cause too many avoidable deaths." *Portland Press Herald*, May 5, 2016.

"Methicillin-resistant Staphylococcus aureus (MRSA) Infections." www.cdc.gov, CDCP, September 16, 2013.

"Mitochondrial Damage and Depletion." www. fluoroquinolonetoxicityofthethyroid.com. June 2017, updated August 2018.

"More Competition for Pharma." *The Wall Street Journal*, May 19, 2018.

"Most adults with bronchitis receive unnecessary antibiotics." *CIDRAP News*, August 25, 2016.

"Nearly 60 percent of patients hospitalized for asthma are prescribed antibiotics." *Weekly Digest*, CDDEP, July 29, 2016.

"New Advice on Treating Sinus Infections With Antibiotics." *Worst Pills Best Pills Newsletter*, August 2012.

"New blood test could help prevrent antibiotic misuse." *PubMedHealth*, March 19, 2015.

"New Evidence That Off-Label Drug Use Increases Risk of Harm." *Worst Pills Best Pills Newsletter*, January 2016.

"New hospital antibiotic stewardship guidelines." *Weekly Digest*, CDDEP, April 17, 2016.

"New Legislation a Windfall for Pharma, False 'Cure' for Patients." www.citizen.org, Public Citizen, December, 2015.

"Often-Misused Fluoroquinolone Antibiotics Pose Serious Risks." *Worst Pills, Best Pills Newsletter*, October 2015.

"Outpatient Quinolone Use." *Weekly Digest*, CDDEP, August 13, 2014.

"Patient Safety Advocates, Industry Spar Over Off-Label Promotion." *Worst Pills Best Pills Newsletter*, January 2017.

"Pharmaceutical Manufacturing/Top Contributors, 2017-2018." www.opensecrets.org.

"Pharmaceuticals/Health Products/Industry Profile: Summary, 2017." www.opensecrets.org.

"Pharma Should Be Open About Money to Patient Groups." www.drugwatch.com.

"Prescriber Report—Systemic Antibiotics." *Drug Store News*, August 29, 2011.

"Protect patients, not patents." *The Economist*, Letter from Medecins San Frontieres Access Campaign, Geneva, January 25, 2014.

"Public Citizen Calls for Black Box Warning on Certain Antibiotics." www.citizen.org, Public Citizen, November 5, 2015.

"Quinolones Market to Undertake Strapping Growth by the End of 2025." *Technology Market*, June 5, 2019.

"QVF Warns of New Fluoroquinolones on the Market." *QVF Newsletter for Summer 2016*, July 31, 2016.

"Reports of adverse events with fluoroquinolones." *FDA Medical Bulletin*, Volume 26, Number 3, October 1996.

"Research Misconduct Identified by the US Food and Drug Administration." *JAMA*, February 9, 2015.

"Researchers develop test to cut overuse of antibiotics." *Portland Press Herald*, September 18, 2013.

"Risk of adverse effecs frm oral antibiotics is higher in young adults." *Weekly Digest*, CDDEP, June 9, 2018.

"Self-prescribing Antibiotics Is A Big Problem." Press release, American Society for Microbiology, July 11, 2016.

"Selling More Drugs by Misrepresenting Their Safety." *Worst Pills Best Pills, Newsletter*, September 2015.

"Settlements for Prosecution of Fraud by Big Pharma

at Record High." *Worst Pills Best Pills Newsletter*, November 2012.

"State Court to Review Cipro Class-Action Lawsuit: AttorneyOne.com Warns the Threat of Severe Adverse Events from Cipro Remains." https://service. pweb.com/pressrelease. March 28, 2012.

"Study Finds Heart Risks with Fluoquinolones." www. drugwatch.com.

"Study: Even one free meal can sway doctors." *Portland Press Herald*, June 21, 2016.

"Sunshine Law Exposes Vast Industry Payments to Physicians." *Worst Pills Best Pills Newsletter*, December, 2014.

"Supreme Court Justice Ginsburg's Drug Interaction Is a Reminder to Pay Attention to Meds." *Worst Pills Best Pills Newsletter*, December 2009.

"Ten Rules for Safer Drug Use." *Worst Pills Best Pills, A Consumer's Guiide to Avoiding Drug-Induced Death or Illness*, Pocket Books, division of Simon & Schuster, Inc., New York, NY. 1990. pp. 864-869.

"Testimony Before the FDA Pediatric Ethics Subcommittee of the Pediatric Advisory Committee by Public Citizen." www.publiccitizen.org, September 9, 2013.

"The 2017 DTC Report: All the data in one place." www. mmm.online.com, Medical Marketing & Media, March 29, 2017.

"The Doctor Will See You (Or Her Screen) Now." *The Wall Street Journal*, Opinion/Letters, May 15, 2016.

"The FDA and Thee." www.wsj.com, November 25, 2013.

"The FDA Should Not Be Promoting Products It Regulates." *Worst Pills Best Pills Newsletter,* November, 2014.

"The Rise of Telemedicine Raises Many Issues." *The Wall Street Journal,* editorial, July 28, 2016.

"Tips to make the most of your doctor visit." *LifeTimes,* Winter 2014.

"Too many antibiotics used in pediatric hospital patients." *Weekly Digest,* CDDEP, April 11, 2018.

"Too Many Meds." *Consumer Reports,* cover story, September 2017.

"U.S. Congressional Legislation Relating to Antibiotic Use, 2004-2014." *GarpNet News,* October, 2014.

"Under patient pressure, antibiotics are more likely to be prescribed, study demonstrates." *Weekly Digest,* CDDEP, February 24, 2017.

"Urinary tract infections (UTIs) in children around the world are highly resistant to common antibiotics." *Weekly Digest,* CDDEP, March 18, 2016.

"Use of antibiotics by prior hospital bed occupants increases risk for *C.difficile* infection in later occupants." *Weekly Digest,* CDDEP, October 14, 2016.

"Vendors in the OR - Veteran Administration's Failed Oversight of Surgical Implants." Subcommittee on Oversight and Investigations (O&I), House of Representatives, Washington, DC . Introductory comments by The Honorable Mike Coffman, Chairman, at subcommittee hearing, January 15, 2014.

"Vital Signs: Improving Antibiotic Use Among Hospitalized Patients; Morbidity and Mortality." *Weekly Report*, CDC, March 7, 2014.

"What Is a Drug Label?" *Worst Pills, Best Pills Newsletter*, June 2016.

"What is a drug product Monograph?" www.globalnews. ca, March 15, 2012.

"What is the most important information I should know about LEVAQUIN? www.levaquin.com.

"What You Need to Know About Fluoroquinolone Antibiotics Like Cipro and Levaquin." www. theheartysoul.com, May 10, 2018.

"When Doctors Don't Listen: How to Avoid Misdiagnoses and Unnecessary Tests." *The Wall Street Journal*, February 19, 2013.

"White House calls for $1.2 billion in antibiotic resistance funding." *Weekly Digest*, CDDEP, January 30, 2015.

Abelson, Reed and Singer, Natasha. "Johnson & Johnson Wins Suit Over Antibiotic's Side Effects." *The New York Times*, October 15, 2011.

Aboubakr, Mohamed et al. "Administration of norfloxacin during pregnancy." *Advances in Pharmacological Sciences*, February 3, 2014.

AbulDagga, Azza, MHA, PhD. "Most Preventive Antibiotics Before Dental Procedures Are Unnecessary, Study Finds." *Health Letter*, December 2019.

Adashi, Eli Y., MD, and Kocher, Robert P., MD. "Physician Self-referral: Regulation by Exceptions." *JAMA*, January 12, 2015.

Airwisan, Adel, et al. "Study Shows that Quinolone Ear Drops Increase Rates of Eardrum Perforation in Children." www.floxiehope.com, April 24, 2017.

Aladdin, Meena, MS, PhD. "Companies Are Reaping Benefits from Social Influencers, and Big Pharma Wants In." *Health Letter*, March 2019.

Almashat, Sammy, MD, MPH, et al. "Rapidly Increasing Criminal and Civil Monetary Penalties Against the Pharmaceutical Industry: 1991 to 2010." Public Citizen Health Research Group report, December 16, 2010.

Almashat, Sammy, MD, MPH. "Medical Journal Editors' Conflicts of Interest Largely Undisclosed." *Health Letter*, Public Citizen, May, 2015.

Almashat, Sammy, MD, MPH. "Pharmaceutical Industry Continues to Defraud Federal, State Governments." *Health Letter*, Public Citizen, April 2016.

Almashat, Sammy, MD, MPH. "Pharmaceutical Lobby Reigns Supreme in Washington." *Health Letter*, Public Citizen, June, 2014.

Almashat, Sammy, MD, MPH. "Pharmaceutical Research Costs: The Myth of the $2.6 Billion Pill." *Health Letter*, Public Citizen, September 2017.

Andriole, Vincent T. "The appropriate use of fluoroquinolones: Factors affecting quinolone use versus other agents: Uses and indications." *Managed Healthcare Executive*, "Considering Your Quinolone Formulary Options" supplement, June, 2002.

Angus, Ian. "Superbugs in the Anthropocene, A Profit-Driven Plague." *Monthly Review*, June 1, 2019.

Arabyat, R.M et al. "Fluoroquinolone-associated tendon-rupture: a summary of reports in the Food and Drug Administration's adverse event reporting system." *PubMed, Epub*, September 22, 2015.

Aspinal, S.L. et al. "Impact of hospital formularies on fluoroquinolone prescribing in emergency departments." *PubMed, Epub*, abstract from *American Journal of Managed Care*, May, 2007.

Asseo, Laurie et al. "Johnson & Johnson to pay $2B in false marketing case." *Chicago Tribune*, November 5, 2013.

Auta, Asa et al. "Global access to antibiotics without prescription in community pharmacies: a systematic review and meta-analysis." *Journal of Infection*, July 5, 2018.

Averch, Timothy D. "Fluoroquinolones: The Emergence of a Toxicity Syndrome." *Urology Practice*, September 2017.

Bakalar, Nicholas. "Antibiotic Use for Sinusitis Is Questioned." *The New York Times*, February 21, 2012.

Bakalar, Nicholas. "Drugs Cause Most Fatal Allergic Reactions, Study Finds." *The New York Times*. October 6, 2014.

Bate, Roger. *Phake, the Deadly World of Falsified and Substandard Medicines*. AEI Press, Washington, DC., 2012.

Bauchner, Howard MD, et al. "Conflicts of Interest, Authors, and Journals. New Challenges for a Persistent Problem." *JAMA*, December 11, 2018.

Bauchner, Howard, MD. "Scientific Misconduct and Medical Journals." *JAMA*, October 20, 2018.

Baumann, Nick. "My Big Levaquin Adventure." *Mother*

Jones, December 7, 2010.

Beck, Melinda. "How Telemedicine Is Transforming Health Care." *The Wall Street Journal,* June 26, 2016.

Beck, Melinda. "Websites Misdiagnose Ailments." *The Wall Street Journal,* May 16, 2016.

Beck, Melinda. "Where Does It Hurt? Log On. The Doctor Is In." *The Wall Street Journal,* May 8, 2014.

Bennett, A. et al. "A Novel Genetic Marker Has Been Identified in Patients With Fluoroquinolone-Associated Neuropsychiatric Toxicity: Preliminary Findings." www.mdedge.com, Association of VA Hematlology/Oncology, AVAHO Updates, Conference Coverage, Abstract 55, August 1, 2017.

Blaser, Martin J. *Missing Microbes: How the Overuse of Antibiotics is Fueling Our Modern Plagues.* Henry Holt and Co., New York, NY, 2014.

Blasi, F. et al. "Highlights on the appropriate use of fluoroquinolones in respiratory tract infections." www. ncbi.nlm.nih.gov/pubmed, abstract from *Pulmonary Pharmacology Therapy*, November 28, 2005 – 2006.

Bloomquist, Lisa. "Don't take Cipro, Levaquin or Avelox if…" www.floxiehope.com, January 27, 2014.

Bloomquist, Lisa. "FDA Announces that Permanent Peripheral Neuropathy is to be Added to Warning Labels for Fluroquinolone Antibiotics." www. floxiehope.com, August 22, 2013.

Bloomquist, Lisa. "The Fluoroquinolone Time Bomb— Answers in the Mitochondria." www.hormonesmatter. com, March 2014.

Boodman, Sandra G. "Diagnosis danger; Experts call for

greater attention to fatal diagnostic errors that happen all the time'." www.chicagotribune.com, *Kaiser Health News*, May 18, 2013.

Boumil, Marcia M., JD, LLM and Curfman, Gregory, MD. "Legal Liability of Generic vs Brand Drug Manufacturers for Inadequate Product Labels," *JAMA*, August 14, 2018.

Bowser, Betty Ann. "Certain Antibiotics Spur Widening Reports of Severe Side Effects." *PBS NewsHour*, June 16, 2011.

Boxer, Richard. "When a Doctor is Always a Phone Call Away." *The Wall Street Journal*, August 2, 2015.

Brill, Steven. "Bitter Pill, Special Report." *Time Magazine*, March 4, 2013.

Brody, Jane E. "A Cure That Can Be Worse Than the Illness." *The New York Times*, September 11, 2012.

Brody, Jane E. "Popular Antibiotics May Carry Serious Side Effects." *The New York Times*, September 10, 2012.

Broniatowski, David et al. "Have a cold? Don't ask your doctor for antibiotics." *The Conversation*, November 25, 2014.

Brummert, Rachel. "QVF Supports Citizen Petition Requesting Another Black Box Warning for Levaquin, Cipro, Avelox. FDA and Drug Makers Asked to Expand Warnings about Psychiatric Adverse Events Risk." www.saferpills.org, Quinolone Vigilance Foundation, November 9, 2014.

Bui, Hoai-Tran. "Antibiotic resistance could be 'next pandemic,' CDC says." *USATODAY*, July 22, 2014.

Burton, Thomas M. "A Low Bar for Some New Antibiotics." *The Wall Street Journal*, March 30, 2014.

Burton, Thomas M. "FDA Panel Recommends Approval of Antibiotics." *The Wall Street Journal*, April 1, 2014.

Burton, Thomas M. "FDA Panel Seeks Tougher Antibiotic Labels." *The Wall Street Journal*, November 5, 2015.

Callaway, Jackie. "Drug maker halts production of antibiotic Levaquin with reported side effects but risk remains." *WFTS*, "ABC Action News," Tampa Bay, FL, October 9, 2018.

Carome, Michael, MD. "Dead Last: U.S. Health Care System Continues to Rank Behind Other Industrialized Countries." *Health Letter*, Public Citizen, November 2014.

Carome, Michael, MD. "New Report Finds Diagnostic Errors Harm 'Unacceptable Number' of Patients." *Health Letter*, Public Citizen, December, 2015.

Carome, Michael, MD. "Outrage of the Month: Doctors Accepting Bribes, Betraying Patients." *Health Letter*, Public Citizen, July 2016.

Carome, Michael, MD. "Outrage of the Month: Ethical Blindness at The New England Journal of Medicine." *Health Letter*, March 2016.

Carome, Michael, MD. "Outrage of the Month: False and Misleading TV Drug Ads." *Health Letter*, Public Citizen, December, 2013.

Carr, Teresa. "Fluoroquinolones Are Too Risky for Common Infections." *Consumer Reports*, May 16, 2016.

Chapman, Steve. "When 'superbugs' outstrip antibiotics."

Chicago Tribune, March 8, 2015.

Cohen, Jay S., MD. "Fluoroquinolone Toxicity Syndrome: A Letter to the Senate Committee on Health, Education & Labor." www.MedicationSense.com, May 9, 2014.

Cohen, Jay S., MD. *What You Must Know About The Hidden Dangers of Antibiotics*, Square One Publishers, Garden City Park, New York, NY, 2018.

Compton, Kristin. "Cipro, Levaquin Elevate Risk for Aortic Aneurysm, Researchers Say." www.drugwatch. com. September 18, 2018.

Connolly, Kevin. "Study Finds Heart Risks with Fluoroquinolones." www.drugwatch.com, March 9, 2018.

Cook, Robin and Topol, Eric. "Cook and Topol: How Digital Medicine Will Soon Save Your Life." *The Wall Street Journal*, February 21, 2014.

Dall, Chris. "Fluoroquinolone stewardship may end at hospital door." *CIDRAP News*, February 13, 2019.

Dallas, Elizabeth March. "Eye-Catching Labels Urged for Fast-Tracked Antibiotics." *HealthDay*, March 2, 2014.

Dameff, Christian, MD et al. "Personal Health Records. More Promising in the Smartphone Era?" www. jamanetwork.com, January 11, 2019.

Daneman, Nick et al. "Fluoroquinolones and collagen associated severe adverse events: a longitudinal cohort study." *CIDRAP News*, November 18, 2015.

Danielson, J. Ryne. "Fluoroquinolones—Mitochondrial Toxicity." www.levaquinadverseeffects.com, April 5, 2015.

Danielson, Ryne. "RX warning: Possible side effects from some antibiotics." *Newsroom*, Medical, University of South Carolina, April 7, 2015.

Davidson, Idelle. "Poisoned: The Dramatic Side Effects of Some Prescription Drugs." *The Washington Post*, August 21, 2015.

Davis, Sallie. Interview on antibiotic overuse, *BBC World News*, June 12, 2013.

Delehanty, Hugh. "Conversation With Sully Sullenberger." *AARP Bulletin*, July-August 2014.

Durkin, Michael et al. "Outpatient Antibiotic Prescription Trends in the United States: A National Cohort Study." *Infection Control & Hospital Epidemiology*, February 27, 2018.

Durkin, Michael et al. "Troubling trend in antibiotic prescriptions in the outpatient setting." www.medicalxpress.com/news, Society for Healthcare Epidemiology of America, March 8, 2018.

Dwoskin, Elizabeth and Walker, Joseph. "Can Data From Your Fitbit Transform Medicine?" *The Wall Street Journal*, June 23, 2014.

Dwoskin, Elizabeth. "The Next Marketing Frontier: Your Medical Records." *The Wall Street Journal*, March 3, 2015.

Eaton, Joe. "Black Market Meds Are Flooding the Nation's Pharmacies and Hospitals." *AARP Bulletin*, May 2016.

Edney, Anna. "FDA head blasts drug supply chain as 'rigged.'" *Portland Press Herald*, March 8, 2018.

Eisler, Peter. "Deadly, drug-resistant bug spreading

beyond hospitals." *USA TODAY,* December 17, 2013.

Evans, Melanie. "Patients Often Get Antibiotics Without a Doctor Visit, Study Finds." *The Wall Street Journal,* February 3, 2020.

Evans, Melanie. "Tech Firms Get Identifiable Hospital Data." *The Wall Street Journal,* January 11, 2020.

Farkas, Josh. "Six reasons to avoid fluoroquinolones in the critically ill." *PulmCrit,* August 1, 2016.

Fassa, Paul. "These Pharmaceutical Antibiotics Can Cause Horrific Side Effects." www.realpharmacy.com, October 16, 2018.

Finn, Holly. "First of All, Get a Second Opinion." *The Wall Street Journal,* March 26, 2013.

Fleming-Dutra, Katherine E., MD et al. "Prevalence of Inappropriate Antibiotic Prescriptions Among US Ambulatory Care Visits, 2010-11." *JAMA,* May 3, 2016.

Frellich, Marcia. "Top 5 New Antibiotics Advance to Fight Resistant Infections." *Medscape Medical News,* October 8, 2018.

Fridkin, MD, et al. "Vital Signs: Improving Antibiotic Use Among Hospitalized Patients." *CDC Morbidity and Mortality Weekly Report,* March 7, 2014.

Fried, Stephen. *Bitter Pills, Inside the Hazardous World of Legal Drugs,* Bantam Books, a division of Random House, New York, NY, 1999.

Fuchs, Victor R., PhD, and Cullen, Mark R., MD. "The Transformation of U.S. Physicians." *JAMA,* May 12, 2015.

Gardner, Caleb and Levinson, John. "Turn Off the Computer and Listen to the Patient." *The Wall Street Journal,* September 21, 2016.

Gawande, Atul, MD, MPH. "The Upgrade." *The New Yorker,* November 12, 2018.

Gellert, George A., MD, MPH, MPA, et al. "The Rise of the Medical Scribe Industry: Implications for the Advancement of Electronic Health Records." *JAMA,* December 15, 2014.

Gerber, Jeffrey S., MD, PhD et al. "Association of Broad vs Narrow Spectrum Antibiotics With Treatment Failure, *Adverse Events,* and Quality of Life in Children With Acute Respiratory Tract Infections." www.jamanetwork.com, December 9, 2017.

Gotzsche, Peter C. *Deadly Medicines and Organised Crime.* Radcliffe Publishing, London, UK, 2013.

Goldacre, Ben. *Bad Pharma: How Drug Companies Mislead Doctors and Harm Patients,* Faber and Faber, New York, NY, 2012.

Goldstein, Jacob. "Lingering Pain from the Anthrax Attacks: Cipro Side Effects." *The Wall Street Journal,* August 7, 2008.

Gough, Alex. "Effect of fluoroquinolone antibiotics on ECGs." *Vet Times,* August 13, 2018.

Gough, Alex. "Effect of fluoroquinolone antibiotics on ECGs." *Vet Times,* August 13, 2018.

Grady, Denise. "Popular Antibiotic May Raise Risk of Sudden Death." *The New York Times,* May 17, 2012.

Graedon, Joe. "A New FDA Warning About Serious Fluoroquinolone Side Effects." *The People's Pharmacy,*

July 12, 2018.

Gribben, Valerie. "Valerie Gribben: Take Two Photos and Call Me in the Morning." *The Wall Street Journal*, August 12, 2013.

Gulfo, Joseph V. "Ending the Prescribe-Don't-Tell Charade for Off-Label Drugs." *The Wall Street Journal*, March 27, 2016.

Haiken, Melanie. "Antibiotic Alert: The Drug The Doctor Ordered Could Cause Deadly Side Effects." *Forbes Magazine*, September 30, 2012.

Hall, Colleen. "Senate Passes Bill to Prohibit Gag Clauses in Pharmacies." *Pharmacy Times*, September 18, 2018.

Hall, M.M et al. "Musculoskeletal complications of fluoroquinolones: guidelines and precautions for usage in the athletic population." *Pub Med, PMR*, February, 2011.

Hamptom, Tracy, PhD. "Optimized Arylomycins May Help Address Antibiotic Resistance." *JAMA*, January 1/8, 2019.

Hampton, Tracy, PhD. "Proposal Seeks to Enhance Availability of Clinical Trial Results." *JAMA*, January 27, 2015.

Healy, David. *Pharmageddon*, University of California Press, Berkeley and Los Angeles, CA, 2012.

Healy, Melissa. "'Slow catastrophe' as golden age of antibiotics nears end." *Los Angeles Times*, July 17, 2016.

Healy, Melissa. "Medication new to the market? Proceed with caution." *Chicago Tribune*, November 11, 2012.

Hilts, Philip J. "F.D.A. Seeks Clear Information Inserts

With Prescription Drugs." *The New York Times*, August 24, 1995.

Hilts, Philip J. *Protecting America's Health; The FDA, Business, and One Hundred Years of Regulation*, University of North Carolina Press, 2004.

Hirschler, Ben and Humer, Caroline. "Drug approvals hit 16-year high in 2012." *Chicago Tribune*, January 1, 2013.

Hirschler, Ben. "Few new antibiotics are in the pipeline. Drugmakers: 'Superbug' threat not widespread enough for costly effort." *Reuters*, London, March 19, 2013.

Hirst, Ellen Jean. "How drugs get their names." *Chicago Tribune*, March 23, 2015.

Hirst, Ellen Jean. "Walgreens app allows virtual visits to doctors." *Chicago Tribune*, December 9, 2014.

Horn, John R., PharmD, FCCP and Hansen, Philip D., PharmD. "Fluoroquinolones and Steroids: An Achilles Heel Interaction." *Pharmacy Times*, April 2016.

Hotz, Robert Lee. "Designing a Hospital to Better Fight Infection." *The Wall Street Journal*, April 27, 2015.

Hotz, Robert Lee. "Scientists Unearth Hope for New Antibiotics." *The Wall Street Journal*, February 12, 2018.

Hudson, Kathy, PhD, et al. "Toward a New Era of Trust and Transparency in Clinical Trials." www.jamanetwork.com, October 4, 2016.

Hughes, Jill Elaine. "Seeking magic in a bottle; Patent medicines promised cures but often delivered dangerous drugs." *Chicago Tribune*, May 5, 2013.

IIgin, Sinew et al. "Ciprofloxacin-induced neurotoxicity: evaluation of possible underlying mechanisms." www. tandmonline.com, *Toxicology Mechanisms and Methods*.

Jena, Anupam B., MD, PhD et al. "The Trade-off Between Speed and Safety in Drug Approvals." *JAMA Oncology*, September 29, 2016.

Joffe, Steven, MD, MPH. "The New Age of Patient Autonomy." www.jamanetwork.org, October 16, 2018.

Johnson, Carolyn Y. "A new worry about antibiotics: Study shows link to mitrochondrial malfunction." *The Boston Globe*, July 8, 2013.

Johnson, Linda A. "FDA names drugmakers accused of blocking cheaper generic drugs." *Portland Press Herald*, *Associated Press*, May 18, 2018

Johnson, Linda A. "J&J stretches diseases initiative." *Chicago Tribune*, March 25, 2016.

Joyner, Michael J MD and Paneth, Nigel MD, MPH. "Seven Questions for Personalized Medicine." *JAMA*, June 22, 2015.

Kaplan, Karen. "Did doctor freebies fuel opiod epidemic? Prescriptions rose as drug companies footed food, travel." *Los Angeles Times*, May 14, 2018.

Kaplan, Sarah. "Some scientists turning to dirt for new source of antibiotics." *Portland Press Herald*, February 14, 2018.

Kavanaugh, Kevin T., MD. "How I Was Prescribed an Unnecessary Antibiotic While Traveling to a Conference on Antibiotic Resistance." *JAMA Internal Medicine*, August 4, 2014.

Klein, Eili. "Does physician competition drive up antibiotic prescribing?" *Weekly Digest*, CDDEP,

January 22, 2015.

Knight, Gwenan M., et al. "Shift in dominant hospital-associated methicillin-resistant *Staphylococcus aureus* clones over time." *Journal of Antimicrobial Chemotherapy*, October 2012, pp. 2514-2522.

Kosova, Weston and Hinman, Kristen. "Princeton Takes Princeton to Court." *Bloomberg Businessweek*, September 23-29.

Kosova, Weston. "The FDA Opens Its Vast Drug Files to the Public." *Bloomberg Businessweek*, March 3-9, 2014.

Kuehn, Bridget M., MSJ. "Patient Safety Still Lagging: Advocates Call for National Patient Safety Monitoring Board." *JAMA*, September 3, 2014.

Lagnado, Lucette. "Are Big Clinical Trials Relevant? Researchers Disagree." *The Wall Street Journal*, May 29, 2018.

Laliberte, Richard. "12 Ways the Heath Care System May Be Harming You." *AARP Bulletin*, September 2016.

Landro, Laura. "A Better Online Diagnosis Before the Doctor Visit." *The Wall Street Journal*, July 22, 2013.

Landro, Laura. "A Medical Detective Story: Why Doctors Make Diagnostic Errors." *The Wall Street Journal*, September 26, 2015.

Landro, Laura. "A Way to Gauge What Your Doctor Knows (or Doesn't)." *The Wall Street Journal*, January 21, 2014.

Landro, Laura. "Hospitals Address a Drug Problem." *The Wall Street Journal*, February 23, 2014.

Landro, Laura. "How Doctors Rate Patients." *The Wall*

Street Journal, March 31, 2014.

Landro, Laura. "How Mainstream Medicine Is Stepping Out of the Mainstream." *The Wall Street Journal*, June 30, 2014.

Landro, Laura. "How Patients Really Can Help Heal Themselves." *The Wall Street Journal*, June 9, 2014.

Landro, Laura. "How to (Really) Get Patients to Take More Control Over Their Medical Decisions."*The Wall Street Journal*, February 27, 2017.

Landro, Laura. "New Tools Help Patients Make Tough Decisions In the ER." *The Wall Street Journal*, April 25, 2016.

Landro, Laura. "Patient 'Passports' Make Sure People With Complex Cases Are Heard." *The Wall Street Journal*, February 2, 2015.

Landro, Laura. "When Doctors Don't Listen: How to Avoid Misdiagnoses and Unnecessary Tests." *The Wall Street Journal*, February 19, 2013.

Landro, Laura."The Doctor's Team Will See You Now." *The Wall Street Journal*, February 17, 2014.

Laue, Tom. "How can time-pressed doctors learn to really hear us?" *LifeTimes*, Winter 2014.

Lawlor, Joe. "Bill targets drug seller payments to doctors." *Portland Press Herald*, January 23, 2017.

Lawlor, Joe. "Pharmacy Middlemen Steer Some Patients to Risker Drugs." *Maine Sunday Telegram*, July 8, 2018.

Laxminarayan, Ramanan. "Antibiotic Resistance." *F&D Financial Development*, December, 2014.

Leitch, Carmen. "The Major HealthRisks Posed by

Cipro." www.labroots.com, August 5, 2018.

Letourneau, Lisa MD. "Five questons to help you 'Choose Wisely' when it comes to health care." *Midcoast Healthy Lifestyles*, Summer 2015.

Levey, Noam N. "Administration cites big decline in medical errors." *Chicago Tribune*, December 3, 2013.

Lewin, Tamar. "A Nation Challenged: Fear of Infections; Anthrax Scare Prompts Run on an Antibiotic." *The New York Times*, September 27, 2001.

Lewis T. and Cook J. "Fluoroquinolones and tendinopathy: a guide for athletes and sports clinicians and a systematic review of the literature." *Pub Med*, *Epub*, April 24, 2014.

Lieber, James B. "How to Make Hospitals Less Deadly." *The Wall Street Journal*, May 17, 2016.

Light, Donald W. "The Epidemic of Sickness and Death from Prescription Drugs." *Footnotes*, November 2014.

Light, Donald W. *The Risks of Prescription Drugs*. Columbia University Press, New York, NY, 2010.

Linder, J.A. et al. "Fluoroquinolone prescribing in the United States: 1995-2002." www.ncbi.nlm.nih.gov/pubmed, abstract from *American Journal of Medicine*, March 2005.

Linder, Jeffrey A., MD, MPH, et al. "Time of Day and the Decision to Prescribe Medicines." *JAMA Internal Medicine*, October 6, 2014.

Loftus, Peter. "Doctors Face New Scrutiny Over Gifts; New Health Law Calls for Increased Disclosures." *The Wall Street Journal*, August 22, 2013.

Loftus, Peter. "Doctors Net Billions From Drug Firms." *The Wall Street Journal*, October 1, 2014.

Loftus, Peter. "Drug Firms Buy Pricey Vouchers to Speed Products to Market." *The Wall Street Journal*, October 20, 2015.

Loftus, Peter. "Even Cheap Meals Influence Doctors' Drug Prescriptions, Study Suggests." *The Wall Street Journal*, June 20, 2016.

Long, Ray and Roe, Sam. "Pharmacy work rules sought to reduce errors." *Chicago Tribune*, February 1, 2017.

Lowes, Robert. "Common Antibiotic Poses Risk to Heart, FDA Warns." *Medscape Medical News*, March 13, 2013.

Lynch, Holly Fernandez, JD, MBE and Joffe, Steven, MD, MPH. "Pay-to-Participate Trials and Vulnerabilities in Research Ethics Oversight." *JAMA*, September 23, 2019.

MacVane, Shawn, PharmD. "Fluoroquinolone Antibiotics: More Recommendations for Prudent Use." *ContagionLive*, October 29, 2018.

Maeder, Thomas. *Adverse Events*, William Morrow and Company, Inc., New York, NY, 1994.

Makary, Marty. "How to Stop Hospitals from Killing Us." *Chicago Tribune*, September 22-23, 2012.

Malone, Patrick and Larson, Anne. "Another Chapter in the Long History of Exposing the Dangers of the Most Popular Drug in America." *Worse Pills Best Pills Newsletter*, July 2009.

Marchant, Jo. "When antibiotics turn toxic." *Nature*, March 21, 2018.

Marcus, Amy Dockser. "New Voices in Medical Advocacy Often Are Patients." *The Wall Streeet Journal*, July 25, 2016.

Martin, Philippe, PhD et al. "Effect of Pharmacist-Led Educational Intervention on Inappropriate Medication Prescriptions in Older Adults." *JAMA*, November 13, 2018.

Martin, S.J. et al. "A risk-benefit assessment of levofloxacin in respiratory, skin and skin structure, and urinary tract infections." Abstract from *Drug Safety*, 2001.

Mathews, Anna Wilde. "Should Doctors and Patients Be Facebook Friends?" *The Wall Street Journal*, February 5, 2013.

Mayne, Sean, MBBS, et al. "Confusion Strongly Associated with Antibiotic Prescribing Due to Suspected Urinary Tract Infections in Nursing Homes." *Journal of the American Geriatrics Society*, January 10, 2018.

McArdle, Megan. "Dealing with Big Pharma rule-breakers." *Chicago Tribune*, January 30, 2015.

McCaffrey, Kevin. "Califf calls for marketers to develop off-label 'code of ethics.'" www.mmm-online.com, Medical Marketing and Media, May 16, 2017.

McCaffrey, Kevin. "PhRMA criticizes the FDA's research into drug advertising and promotion." www.mmm-online.com, Medical Marketing and Media, August 17, 2017.

McCaughey, Betsey. "When Hospitals Become Killers." *The Wall Street Journal*, January 31, 2013.

McKay, Betsy and Bauerlein, Valerie. "CDC: Antibiotic

Overuse Can Be Lethal." *The Wall Street Journal,* March 4, 2014.

McKay, Betsy. "Antibiotics Losing Battle Against Bugs: Report." *The Wall Street Journal,* September 16, 2013.

McKay, Betsy. "New Push to Stop Overuse of Antibiotics in Nursing Homes." *The Wall Street Journal,* October 12, 2015.

Meikle, James. "Doctors write 10m needless antibiotics prescriptions a year, says NICE." www.theguardian.com/society, August 18, 2015.

Michalak, K. et al. "Treatment of the Fluoroquinolone-Associated Disability: The Pathobiochemical Implications." www.ncbi.nim.nih.gov, *PubMed, Epub,* September 2017.

Miller, Henry I. "Critics of 'Me-Too Drugs' Need to Take a Chill Pill." *The Wall Street Journal,* January 1, 2014.

Minsky, Bonnie, MA, MPH, LDN, DNS and Minsky, Steve. "Probiotics just as good as antibiotics for UTIs." www.nutritionalconcepts.blogspot.com, May 23, 2012.

Minsky, Bonnie, MA, MPH, LDN, DNS. "Disturbing New Developments With Antibiotic, Bone Drugs." *NCI Well Connect Mid-Week Brief,* August 21, 2013.

Minsky, Bonnie, MA, MPH, LDN, DNS. "Do Docs & Nurses Take Supplements?" *NCI Well Connect Newsletter,* January 7, 2019.

Minsky, Steve. "Shame on This Hospital Policy." www.nutritionalconcepts.com. *NCI Well Connect Newsletter,* June 13, 2016.

Monti, Adrian. "Common antibiotic doctors say could

give you organ failure as millions of Britons are at risk of devastating permanent side effect as a result of over-prescribing." *Daily Mail*, October 27, 2018.

Moreno, Jonathan D., PhD et al. "The Nuremberg Code 70 Years Later." *JAMA*, September 5, 2017.

Moyers, Bill. "Interview with Melody Petersen." www.pbs. org/moyers/Journal, May 16, 2008.

Mulvey, Michael R., PhD and Simor, Andrew E., MD. "Antimicrobial resistance in hospitals: How concerned should we be?" *CMAJ*, February 17, 2009.

Muto, Carlene A., MD et al. "A Large Outbreak of Clostridium Difficile-Associated Disease With an Unexpected Proportion of Deaths and Colectomies at a Teaching Hospital Following Increased Fluoroquinolone Use." *Infecton Control and Hospital Epidemiology*, March 2005.

Nambudiri, Vinod E., MD, MBA. "More Than Skin Deep—The Costs of Antibiotic Overuse." *JAMA Internal Medicine*, September 1, 2014.

Nesi, Tom. *Poison Pills, the Untold Story of the Vioxx Drug Scandal.* St. Martin's Press, New York, NY, 2008.

Newkirk, Margaret and Berfield, Susan. "How Do You Stop Taking Recalled Medication If You Don't Know It's Been Recalled?" *Bloomberg Businessweek*, December 13, 2019.

Noah, Timothy. "The Make-Believe Billion; How drug companies exaggerate research costs to justify absurd profits." www.slate.com, *Slate Magazine*.

O'Connor, Jim. "Drugs advertised on television contribute to high medical costs." *Portland Press*

Herald, August 3, 2014.

Ornstein, Charles et al. "As sunshine law nears, Big Pharma trims." *Chicago Tribune*, March 5, 2014.

Ornstein, Charles et al. "We Found Over 700 Doctors Who Were Paid More than a Million Dollars by Drug and Medical Device Companies." www.propublica.org, October 17, 2019.

Ornstein, Charles. "Cipro recipients developing side effects." *Chicago Tribune*, November 9, 2001.

Ortiz, Selena E., MPH and Rosenthal, Meredith B., PhD. "Medical Marketing, Trust, and the Patient-Physician Relationship." *JAMA*, January 8, 2019.

Ostrow, Nicole. "U.S. Nonprofit Hospital CEO Annual Pay Averages $600,000." *Bloomberg*, October 14, 2013.

Painter, Kim. "1 in 25 hospital patients get an infection during care." *USA TODAY*, March 27, 2014.

Panas, Marios, MD, PhD. "Hereditary Neuropathy Unmasked by Levofloxacin." *The Annals of Pharmacotherapy*, August 31, 2011.

Park, Alice. "A Cautionary Tale About Antibiotics." *Time Magazine*, April 14, 2016.

Park, Alice. "Antibiotics Are Still Overused in Hospitals." *Time Magazine*, September 19, 2016.

Parker-Pope, Tara. "Antibiotics Like Cipro Are Linked to Tendon, Psychiatric Problems." *The Wall Street Journal*, October 26, 2001.

Parker-Pope, Tara. "Overtreatment Is Taking a Harmful Toll." *The New York Times*, August 27, 2012.

Parker-Pope, Tara. "Surge in Use of Cipro Spurs Concerns About Side Effects." *The Wall Street Journal,* October 26, 2001.

Parsa-Parsi, Ramin Walter, MD, MPH. "The Revised Declaration of Geneva. A Modern-Day Physician's Pledge." *JAMA,* November 28, 2017.

Paturel, Amy. "How to talk so your doctor will listen." *AARP Bulletin,* January-February 2017.

Perryman, Dr. John. "Pharma fallacies." *Chicago Tribune,* January 11, 2018.

Petersen, Melody. *Our Daily Meds: How the Pharmaceutical Companies Transformed Themselves into Slick Marketing Machines and Hooked the Nation on Prescription Drugs.* Picador, New York, NY. 2008.

Pettypiece, Shannon. "Drug merger could mean lab closings, less research." *Chicago Tribune,* May 2, 2014.

Piller, Charles. "FDA and NIH let clinical trial sponsors keep results secret, investigation shows." *Science Magazine,* January 2020.

Ping-Hsun, Wu. "Risk of gastrointestinal perforation in patients taking oral fluoroquinolone therapy." *PLOS One,* September 5, 2017.

Plumridge, Hester. "Drug Makers Tiptoe Back Into Antibiotic R&D." *The Wall Street Journal,* January 23, 2014.

Powell, Alvin. "The threat from superbugs; Panel says dangers from increasingly ineffective antibiotics continue to rise." www.news.harvard.edu, Harvard Gazette, February 9, 2014.

Preidt, Robert. "FDA Adds Stronger Warnings to

Fluoroquinolones." www.webmd.com, July 11, 2018.

Pronovost, Peter. "How to Keep Doctors From Overprescribing Antibiotics." *The Wall Street Journal*, June 30, 2017.

Ranaivo, Yann. "UAB researchers: Inappropriate antibiotics use in ERs still a problem." *Birmingham Business Journal*, January 22, 2014.

Rapaport, Lisa. "Common medicines tied to changes in the brain." *Reuters*, April 20, 2016.

Rapp, Adam. "10 Big Pharma Statistics That Will Make You Cringe." www.emedcert.com, July 13, 2016.

Rappoport, Jon. "Why the FDA should be charged with murder." www.nomorefakenews.com, May 16, 2014.

Ray, Kristin N. et al. "Antibiotic Prescribing During Pediatric Direct-to-Consumer Telemedicine Visits." *Pediatrics*, April 2019.

Reddy, Sumathi. "Antibiotics Do's and Don'ts." *The Wall Street Journal*, August 20, 2013.

Reddy, Sumathi. "Drugstores Play Doctor: Physicals, Flu Diagnosis and More." *The Wall Street Journal*, April 7, 2014.

Reddy, Sumathi. "New Thinking on Sinus Infections." *The Wall Street Journal*, April 6, 2015.

Reddy, Sumathi. "Side Effects: Telling the Real From the Imagined." *The Wall Street Journal*, July 7, 2014.

Reddy, Sumathi. "The Question of When to Stop Antibiotics." *The Wall Street Journal*, August 15, 2017.

Reddy, Sumathi. "When Patients Are a Pain for Their Doctors." *The Wall Street Journal*, April 4, 2016.

Redford, Gabrielle. "Conversation With Francis Collins, director of the National Institutes of Health." *AARP Bulletin*, March 2014.

Reilly, Brendan. "Give It To Me Straight, Doc." *The Wall Street Journal*, March 14, 2016.

Reviglio, Victor E. et al. "Effect of topical fluroquinolones on the expression of matrix metalloproteinases in the cornea." *BMC Ophthalmology*, October 6, 2003.

Ricks, Delthia. "CDC urges caution on antibiotics." *Chicago Tribune*. December 4, 2013.

Roberts, Rebecca, MS et al. "Variation in US Outpatient Antibiotic Prescribing." www.ajmc.com/journals, August 17, 2016.

Robertson, Jordan. "Your Not-So-Secret Medical History." *Bloomberg Businessweek*, August 8-12, 2013.

Robotti, Suzanne B. "Floxed! The Painful, Life-Lasting Effects of Some Antibiotics." www.medshadow.org, April 3, 2018.

Rockoff, Jonathan D. "J&J Hires Chief Design Officer." *The Wall Street Journal*, March 19, 2014.

Rockoff, Jonathan D. "Knockoffs of Biotech Drugs Bring Paltry Savings." *The Wall Street Journal*, May 5, 2016.

Rockoff, Jonathan D. and Loftus, Peter. "Branded Drugs Chalk Up a Win Under Health Law." *The Wall Street Journal*, November 3, 2013.

Rockoff, Jonathan D. and Plumridge, Hester. "Drug Firms Curb Ties to Doctors." *The Wall Street Journal*, December 17, 2013.

Rockoff, Jonathan D. and Silverman, Ed. "Pharmaceutical

Companies Buy Rivals' Drugs, Then Jack Up the Prices." *The Wall Street Journal*, April 26, 2015.

Rockoff. Jonathan D. "The Big Business of Orphan Drugs." *The Wall Street Journal*, January 31, 2013.

Rodriguez, Tori. "Essential Oils Might Be the New Antibiotics." *The Atlantic*, January, 2015.

Roe, Sam and Long, Ray. "Pharmacy chains improve drug alerts." *Chicago Tribune*, August 9, 2017.

Roe, Sam et al. "Filled without warning." *Chicago Tribune*, December 18, 2016.

Rosenberg, Martha. *Born with a Junk Food Deficiency: How Flaks, Quacks, and Hacks Pimp the Public Health*, Prometheus Books, Amherst NY, 2012.

Rubin, Rita, MA. "FDA Fails to Adequately Track Safety of Expedited Drugs." www.jamanetwork.org, March 8, 2016.

Russell, John. "One Drug Nine Uses." *Chicago Tribune*, September 20, 2015.

Saboo, Alok and Palmer, Eric. "The top 10 pharma companies by 2013 revenue. www.fiercepharma.com, March 4, 2014.

Sadick, Barbara. "A Push for Less Testing in Emergency Rooms." *The Wall Street Journal*, February 23, 2014.

Sadick, Barbara. "Physician Burnout." *Chicago Tribune*, October 22, 2014.

Sadick, Barbara. "The Hospital Room of the Future." *The Wall Street Journal*, November 17, 2013.

Savage, David G. "High court to rule on 'pay for delay' deals." *Chicago Tribune*, December 9, 2012.

Schulte, Fred and Fry, Erika. "Electronic Health Records Creating a 'New Era' of Health Care Fraud, Officials Say." *Fortune*, December 23, 2019.

Schwartz, Lisa M. and Woloshin, Steven. "The Drug Facts Box: Improving the communication of prescription drug information." *Procedures of the National Academy of Science USA*, August 20, 2013.

Seife, Charles, MS. "Research Misconduct Identified by the US Food and Drug Administration, Out of Sight, Out of Mind, Out of the Peer-Reviewed Literature." *JAMA*, February 9, 2015.

Sharfstein, Joshua M., MD et al. "The Promotion of Medical Products in the 21st Century: Off-label Marketing and First Amendment Concerns." *JAMA*, September 14, 2015.

Sharpe, Katherine. "Medication: The smart-pill oversell." *Nature*, February 12, 2014.

Shaywitz, David A. "Doctor Android; In the same way that Luther challenged the Catholic Church, smartphones are poised to upend the medical profession." *The Wall Street Journal*, January 12, 2015.

Silverman, Ed. "Levaquin Causes A 'Lot of Damage' Fratti Explains." www.pharmalot.com. February 23, 2012.

Silverman, Ed. "Sharing Some Clinical Trial Data Remains a Problem for Pharma." *The Wall Street Journal*, January 29, 2014.

Silvestrini, Elaine. "Study Finds Heart Risks with Fluoroquinolones." www.drugwatch.com, March 9, 2018.

Singh, Hardeep, Dr. "The Battle Against Misdiagnosis:

American doctors make the wrong call more than 12 million times a year." *The Wall Street Journal*, August 7, 2014.

Sinha, Michael S., MD, JD, MPH et al. "Antitrust, Market Exclusivity, and Transparency in the Pharmaceutical Industry." *JAMA*, May 7, 2018.

Skarecky, Douglas et al. "Fluoroquinolones: The Emergence of a Toxicity Syndrome." *Urology Practice*, September 2017.

Sorscher, Sarah, JD, MPH. "Cures for the 21st Century: Five Simple Ideas Congress Has Ignored." *Health Letter*, Public Citizen, April 2015.

Southey, Flora. "EMA risk committee recommends quinolone antibiotics be removed from market." www.inpharmatechnologist.com. October 22, 2018.

Spatz, Erica S., MD, MHS et al. "The New Era of Informed Consent. Getting to a Reasonable-Patient Standard Through Shared Decision Making." *JAMA*, May 17, 2016.

Specter, Michael. "The Operator; Is the most trusted doctor in America doing more harm than good?" *The New Yorker*, February 4, 2013.

Staton, Tracy. "A new wave of Levaquin lawsuits, patients claim J&J knew about nerve-damage risks." *FiercePharma*, August 16, 2016.

Stiegler, Marjorie Podraza, MD. "What I Learned About Adverse Events From Captain Sully." *JAMA*, January 27, 2015.

Sugarman, Deborah Tolmach, MSW, and Jin, Jill, MD, MPH. "Talking to Your Doctor About Tests, Treatments, and Their Costs." *JAMA*, November 26,

2014.

Sun, Lena H. "1 in 3 antibiotics prescribed in U.S. are unnecessary, major study finds." *The Washington Post*, May 3, 2016.

Sun, Lena H. "Hospital antibiotic use can put patients at risk, study says." *Health & Science*, March 4, 2014.

Sun, Lena H. "Patients often get wrong diagnoses from doctors, report finds." *Chicago Tribune*, September 23, 2015.

Sun, Lena H. "Study: Clinics prescribing antibiotics too often." *Portland Press Herald*, July 17, 2018.

Sutcliffe, Kathleen. "How to Reduce Medical Errors." *Time Magazine*, November 25, 2019.

Tamma, Pranita D., MD, MHS and Cosgrove, Sara E., MD, MS. "Addressing the Appropriateness of Outpatient Antibiotic Prescribing in the United States." *JAMA*, May 3, 2016.

Tamma, Pranita D., MD, MHS et al. "Rethinking How Antibiotics Are Prescribed." www.jamanetwork.com, December 27, 2018.

Tanner, Lindsey. "Medical marketing hits $30B." *Chicago Tribune*, January 10, 2019.

Theuretzbacher, Ursula. "Recent FDA Antibiotic Approvals: Good News and Bad News." *Weekly Digest*, CDDEP, March 12, 2015.

Thomas, Helen. "Beware the Thundering Pharma Herd." *The Wall Street Journal*, January 5, 2014.

Thurston, Andrew, MD. "The Unreasonable Patient." www.jamanetwork.org, February 16, 2016.

Tobacman, Jessica. "FDA alerts record mixed, U. of C. study finds." *Chicago Tribune*, February 15, 2012.

Tomlinson, Kathy. "Pharmacists' failure to check drug risks leads to 'horrible' death." *CBC News*, October 6, 2014.

Topol, Eric. "Eric Topol on the Future of Medicine." *The Wall Street Journal*, July 7, 2014.

Tozzi, John. "The FDA Opens Its Vast Drug Files to the Public." *Bloomberg Businessweek*, March 3-March 9, 2014.

Van Eschenback, Andrew. "Toward a 21st-Century FDA." *Chicago Tribune*. April 16, 2012.

Volker, Rebecca, MSJ. "Another Fluoroquinolone Approved." www.jamanetwork.com, August 1, 2017.

Voreacos, David and Decker, Susan. "Princeton Takes Princeton to Court; Residents want a piece of the school's millions in patent income; some faculty are becoming fabulously wealthy." *Bloomberg Businessweek*, September 23-29, 2013.

Vosovic, Aleksandar and Hirschler, Ben. "Bribery infections spreading; Probes by U.S., British regulators target alleged rise of illicit payments to doctors in emerging markets." *Chicago Tribune*, March 1, 2012.

Walker, Joseph. "Drug Industry Launches Ad Campaign Aimed at Lawmakers." *The Wall Street Journal*, February 7, 2016.

Walker, Joseph. "FDA Advisers' Financial Ties Not Disclosed." *The Wall Street Journal*, December 8, 2014.

Walker, Joseph. "How FDA Assembles Advisory Panels."

www.wsj.com, December 8, 2014.

Wang, Shirley S. "Antibiotics of the Future." *The Wall Street Journal*, December 16, 2013.

Washington, Harriet A. *Deadly Monopolies, the Shocking Corporate Takeover of Life Itself—and the Consequences for Your Health and Our Medical Future*. Anchor Books, Random House, New York, NY, November 2012.

Wasserman, Emily. "Levaquin users slap J&J with $800M RICO suit, claiming pharma giant hid serious side effects." www.fiercepharma.com, January 21, 2016.

Wasson, Julia. "Indie Film Describes 'Certain Adverse Events' from Antibiotic Use," www.organicgreenandnatural.com, August 31, 2009.

Werner, Nicole L., et al. "Unnecessary use of fluroquinolone antibiotics in hospitalized patients." www.biomedcentral.com July 5, 2011.

Werth, Barry. "Tale of Two Drugs." *MIT Technology Review*, November/December 2013.

Whalen, Jeanne. "Health-Care Apps That Doctors Use." *The Wall Street Journal*, November 17, 2013.

Wilcox, Jennifer. "The Road to Recovery After a Side Effect Changed One Woman's Life." www.news.goraw.com, March 20, 2014.

Wilensky, Gail, PhD. "Changing Physician Behavior Is Harder Than We thought." *JAMA*, July 5, 2016.

Willman, David. "Pointing to threat, pulling in profit; Pentagon adviser touted anti-anthrax drug—and was on drugmaker's board." *Chicago Tribune*, May 19, 2013.

Wolfe, Sidney M., MD. "Crime in the Pharma Suites." *Health Letter,* Public Citizen, June 2010.

Wolfe, Sidney M., MD. "Dangers of Overdiagnosis and Overtreatment." *Health Letter,* Public Citizen, March 2012.

Wolfe, Sidney M., MD. "Don't Get Sick in July." *Health Letter,* Public Citizen, August 2010.

Wolfe, Sidney M., MD. "For Big Pharma, Crime Pays." *Health Letter,* Public Citizen, November 2011.

Wolfe, Sidney M., MD. "More About Drug Industry Lawlessness." *Health Letter,* Public Citizen, February 2013.

Wolfe, Sidney, M., MD. "FDA Must Do More to Warn Patients Taking Fluoroquinolone Antibiotics of Possible Tendon Ruptures." www.citizen.org, Press Room, July 8, 2008.

Wolfe, Sidney, M., MD. "FDA's Drug Review Process is Broken." 2014 Shine Lecture by Dr. Wolfe at the Boston University School of Public Health, March 5, 2014.

Wolfe, Sidney, M., MD. "More Despicable Drug-Industry Behavior." *Health Letter,* Public Citizen, December 2011.

Wolfe, Sidney, M., MD. "Patient Advocacy Groups and Drug Company Funding." *Health Letter,* Public Citizen, April 211.

Xu, Tim, MPP et al. "The Potential Hazards of Hospital Consolidation: Implications for Quality, Access and Price." *JAMA,* August 13, 2015.

Yang, Guang et al. "Tendon and Ligament Regeneration and Repair: Clinical Relevance and Developmental

Paradigm." HHS Public Access, National Institute of Health, June 2, 2014.

Young, Robin and Hobson, Jeremy. "The Search For New Antibiotics." National Public Radio, February 17, 2014.

Zang Kun. "The Growing Resistance to Antibiotics." *Beyond Beijing*, May 15, 2014.

Zinberg, Joel, MD. "Physicians who are employees of hospitals will split their allegiances between their employers and patients." *The Wall Street Journal,* December 22, 2014.

Zweig, Phillip L. and Blum, Frederick C. "Where Does the Law Against Kickbacks Not Apply? Your Hospital." *The Wall Street Journal,* May 7, 2018.

INDEX

Achilles tendon
2, 6-7, 20-22, 25, 79

adverse effect
12, 18, 20, 24, 36, 44, 45, 76, 78, 84, 92, 98, 114, 119, 122, 131, 145, 146, 152

adverse event
7, 19, 24, 44, 47-48, 77-78, 86, 201, 130, 141, 143, 152

advertising
24, 37, 43, 49-50, 53-54, 62, 64, 86, 103, 105, 107, 130

advocacy
109, 134, 150, 153

Agency for Healthcare Research and Quality
(AHRQ)
122

aneurysm
21, 82

anthrax
84

antibiotic resistance
29, 63, 91, 98 141, 151, 188

antibiotics
3, 5, 10, 11, 16, 18, 21, 23, 28, 30, 36, 38, 40, 43, 72, 75, 81, 91-94 96-99, 104, 115, 118-123, 125, 130, 133, 140-143, 147, 149, 150-151, 154

applications for drug approval
40, 72, 74-75

www.ingramcontent.com/pod-product-compliance
Lightning Source LLC
Chambersburg PA
CBHW052128270326
41930CB00012B/2796